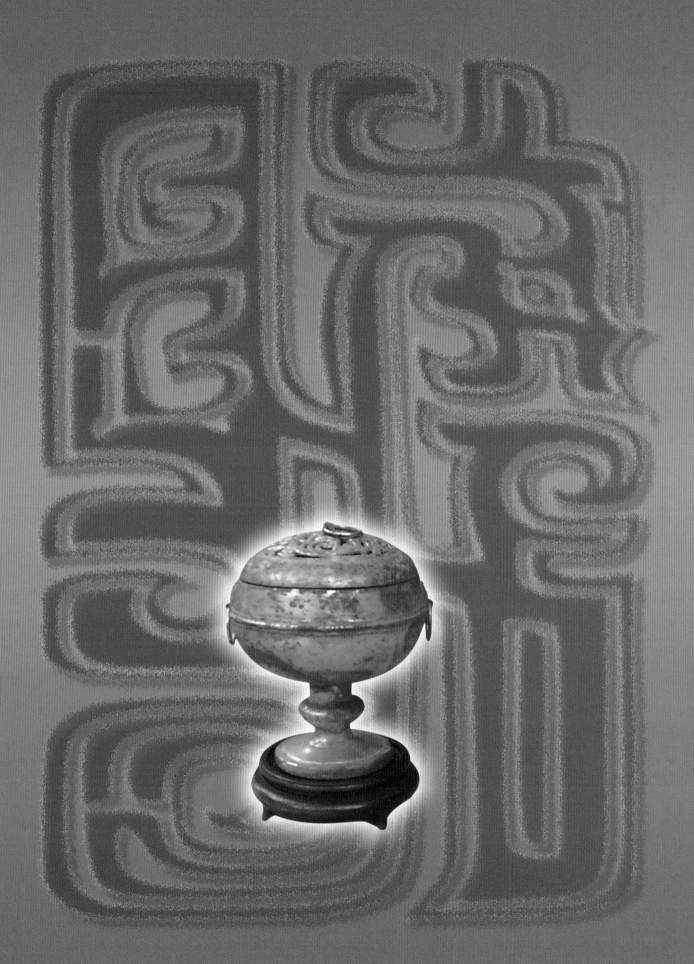

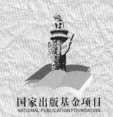

国家出版基金项目
NATIONAL PUBLICATION FOUNDATION

中华医药卫生

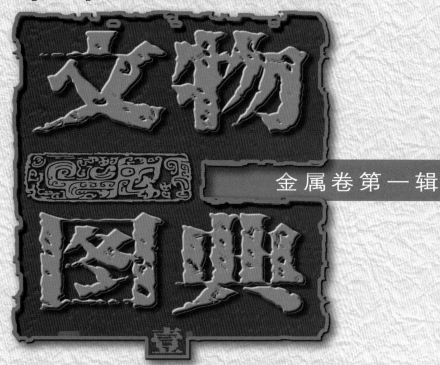

金属卷第一辑

主　编　李经纬　梁　峻　刘学春
总主译　白永权
主　译　聂文信

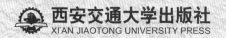

西安交通大学出版社
XI'AN JIAOTONG UNIVERSITY PRESS

图书在版编目 (CIP) 数据

中华医药卫生文物图典 . 1. 金属卷 . 第 1 辑 . / 李经纬，
梁峻，刘学春主编 .— 西安：西安交通大学出版社，2016.12

ISBN 978-7-5605-7023-5

Ⅰ . ①中… Ⅱ . ①李… ②梁… ③刘… Ⅲ . ①中国医药学—
金属器物—古器物—中国—图录 Ⅳ . ① R-092 ② K870.2

中国版本图书馆 CIP 数据核字（2015）第 013550 号

书　　名　中华医药卫生文物图典（一）金属卷第一辑

主　　编　李经纬　梁　峻　刘学春

责任编辑　李　晶　张沛烨

出版发行　西安交通大学出版社
　　　　　（西安市兴庆南路 10 号　邮政编码 710049）

网　　址　http://www.xjtupress.com

电　　话　（029）82668805 82668502（医学分社）
　　　　　（029）82668315（总编办）

传　　真　（029）82668280

印　　刷　中煤地西安地图制印有限公司

开　　本　889mm×1194mm　1/16　印张 36.25　字数 575 千字

版次印次　2017 年 12 月第 1 版　2017 年 12 月第 1 次印刷

书　　号　ISBN 978-7-5605-7023-5

定　　价　1080.00 元

读者购书、书店添货、如发现印装质量问题，请通过以下方式联系、调换。

订购热线：（029）82665248　（029）82665249

投稿热线：（029）82668805　（029）82668502

读者信箱：medpress@126.com

銘記感受歷史

自信自重自強

書賀

中華醫藥衛生文物圖典問世

陳可冀 二〇一七年春日 謹題

陈可冀　中国科学院院士、国医大师

精修醫藥衛生文物

圖典功著當代

深究岐黃學術思想

淵源惠澤千秋

中華醫藥衛生文物圖典出版誌慶

丁酉孟秋 孫光榮 敬題於北京

孙光荣　国医大师

中華醫藥衛生文物圖典出版

彰顯中醫藥
文化精神

體現中醫藥
歷史價值

歲次丁酉夏 王琦

王琦 国医大师

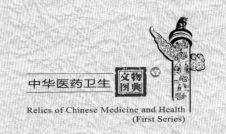

中华医药卫生
Relics of Chinese Medicine and Health
(First Series)

中华医药卫生文物图典（一）
丛书编撰委员会

主　编　李经纬　梁　峻　刘学春

副主编　廖　果　吴鸿洲　康兴军　和中浚　刘小斌　杨金生

　　　　　郑怀林　徐江雁　白建疆　黄　煌

编　委　李洪晓　梁永宣　王强虎　董树平　马　健　王　霞

　　　　　张雅宗　朱德明　包哈申　张建青　郑　蓉　庄乾竹

　　　　　李宏红　刘哲峰　王宏才　陈润东

总主译　白永权

主　译　陈向京　聂文信　范晓晖　温　睿　赵永生　杜彦龙

　　　　　吉　乐　李小棉　郭　梦　陈　曦

副主译（按姓氏音序排列）

　　　　　董艳云　姜雨孜　李建西　刘　慧　马　健　任宝磊

　　　　　任　萌　任　莹　王　颇　习通源　谢皖吉　徐素云

　　　　　许崇钰　许　梅　詹菊红　赵　菲　邹郝晶

译 者（按姓氏音序排列）

迟征宇　邓　甜　付一豪　高　琛　高　媛　郭　宁

韩　蕾　何宗昌　胡勇强　黄　鋆　蒋新蕾　康晓薇

李静波　刘雅恬　刘妍萌　鲁显生　马　月　牛笑语

唐云鹏　唐臻娜　田　多　铁红玲　佟健一　王　晨

王　丹　王　栋　王　丽　王　媛　王慧敏　王梦杰

王仙先　吴耀均　席　慧　肖国强　许子洋　闫红贤

杨姣姣　姚　晔　张　阳　张　鋆　张继飞　张梦原

张晓谦　赵　欣　赵亚力　郑　青　郑艳华　朱江嵩

朱瑛培

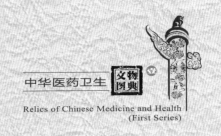

中华医药卫生 文物图典

Relics of Chinese Medicine and Health
(First Series)

本册编撰委员会

主　编　李经纬　梁　峻　刘学春

副主编　廖　果　吴鸿洲　康兴军　和中浚　刘小斌　杨金生
　　　　郑怀林　徐江雁　白建疆　黄　煌

编　委　李洪晓　梁永宣　王强虎　董树平　马　健　王　霞
　　　　张雅宗　朱德明　包哈申　张建青　郑　蓉　庄乾竹
　　　　李宏红　刘哲峰　王宏才　陈润东

总主译　白永权

主　译　聂文信

副主译　吉　乐

译　者　王慧敏　迟征宇　张梦原　高　琛　王　媛　唐臻娜
　　　　牛笑语　吴耀均　黄　鍪　蒋新蕾　席　慧　姜雨孜

丛书策划委员会

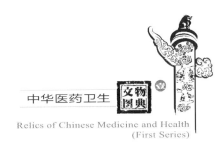

序　言

　　探索天、地、人运动变化规律以及"气化物生"过程的相互关系，是人类永恒的课题。宇宙不可逆，地球不可逆，人生不可逆业已成为共识。天地造化形成自然，人类活动构成文化。文物既是文化的载体，又是物化的历史，还是文明的见证。

　　追求健康长寿是人类共同的夙愿。中华民族之所以繁衍昌盛，健康文化起了巨大的推动作用。由于古人谋求生存发展、应对环境变化产生的智慧，大多反映在以医药卫生为核心的健康文化之中，所以，习总书记说："中医药学是中国古代科学的瑰宝，也是打开中华文明宝库的钥匙"。

　　秉持文化大发展、大繁荣理念，中国中医科学院李经纬、梁峻等为负责人的科研团队在完成科技部"国家重点医药卫生文物收集调研和保护"课题获 2005 年度中华中医药学会科技二等奖基础上，又资鉴"夏商周断代工程""中华文明探源工程"等相关考古成果，用有重要价值的新出土文物置换原拍摄质量较差的文物，适当补充民族医药文物，共精选收载 5000 余件。经西安交通大学出版社申报，《中华医药卫生文物图典（一）》（以下简称《图典》）于 2013 年获得了国家出版基金的资助，并经专业翻译团队翻译，使《图典》得以面世。

　　文物承载的信息多元丰富，发掘解读其中蕴藏的智慧并非易事。　医药卫生文物更具有特殊性，除文物的一般属性外，还承载着传统医学发展史迹与促进健康的信息。运用历史唯物主义观察发掘文物信息，善于从生活文物中领悟卫生信息，才能准确解读其功能，也才能诠释其在民生健康中的历史作用，收到以古鉴今之效果。"历史是现实的根源"，任何一个民族都不能割断历史，史料都包含在文化中。"文化是民族的血脉，是人民的精神家园"，文化繁荣才能实现中华民族的伟大复兴。值本《图典》付梓之际，用"梳理文化之脉，必获健康之果"作为序言并和作者、读者共勉！

中央文史研究馆馆员
中国工程院院士　王永炎
丁酉年仲夏

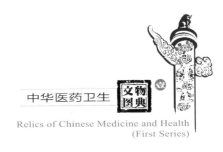

中华医药卫生 文物图典

Relics of Chinese Medicine and Health
(First Series)

前 言

　　文化是相对自然的概念，是考古界常用词汇。文物是文化的重要组成部分，既是文明的物证，又是物化的历史。狭义医药卫生文物是疾病防治模式语境下的解读，而广义医药卫生文物则是躯体、心态、环境适应三维健康模式下的诠释。中华民族是 56 个民族组成的多元一体大家庭，中华医药卫生文物当然包括各民族的健康文化遗存。

　　天地造化如造山、板块漂移、气候变迁、生物起源进化等形成自然。气化物生莫贵于人，即整个生物进化的最高成果是人类自身。广义而言，人类生存思维留下的痕迹即物质财富和精神财富总和构成文化，其一般的物化形式是视觉感知的文物、文献、胜迹等。其中质变标志明晰的文化如文字、文物、城市、礼仪等可称作文明。从唯物史观视角观察，狭义文化即精神财富，尤其体现人类精、气、神状态的事项，其本质也具有特殊物质属性，如量子也具有波粒二相性，这种粒子也是物质，无非运动方式特殊而已。现代所谓可重复验证的"科学"，事实上也是从文化中分离出来的事项，因此也是一种特殊文化形式。追求健康长寿是人类共同的夙愿。中华民族之所以繁衍昌盛，是因为健康文化异彩纷呈。中华优秀传统医药文化之所以博大精深，是因为其原创思维博大、格物致知精深，所以，习总书记说："中医药学是中国古代科学的瑰宝，也是打开中华文明宝库的钥匙"。

文化既反映时代、地域、民族分布、生产资料来源、技术水平等信息，又反映人类认知水平和生存智慧。发掘解读文物、文献中蕴藏的健康知识和灵动智慧，首先是从事健康工作者的责任和义务。《易经》设有"观"卦，人类作为观察者，不仅要积极收藏展陈文物，而且要善于捕捉文物倾诉的信息，汲取养分，启迪思维，收到古为今用之效果。墨子三表法，首先一表即"本之于古者圣王之事"，也是强调古代史实的重要性。"历史是现实的根源"，现实是未来的基础。任何一个国家、地区、民族都不能割断历史、忽略基础，这个基础就是文化。"文化是民族的血脉，是人民的精神家园"。文化繁荣才能驱动各项事业发展，才能实现中华民族的伟大复兴。

人类从类人猿分化出来。"禄丰古猿禄丰种"是云南禄丰发现的类人猿化石，距今七八百万年。距今 200 万年前人类进入旧石器时代，直立行走，打制石器产生工具意识，管理火种，是所谓"燧人氏"时代。中国留存有更新世早、中期的元谋、蓝田、北京人等遗址。距今 10 万—5 万年前，人类进入旧石器时代中期，即早期智人阶段，脑容量增加，和欧洲、非洲人种相比，原始蒙古人种颧骨前突等，是所谓"伏羲氏"时代。中国发现的马坝、长阳、丁村人等较典型。距今 5 万—1 万年前，人类进入旧石器时代晚期，即晚期智人阶段，细石器、骨角器等遍布全国，山顶洞、柳江、资阳人等较典型。

中石器时代距今约 1 万年，是旧石器时代向新石器时代的短暂过渡期，弓箭发明，狗被驯化。河南灵井、陕西沙苑遗址等作为代表。距今 1 万一公元前 2600 年前后，人类进入新石器时代，磨光石器、烧制陶器，出现农业村落并饲养家畜，是所谓"神农氏"时代。公元前 7000 年以来，在甲、骨、陶、石等载体上出现契刻符号、七音阶骨笛乐器等，反映出人文气息趋浓。公元前 6000—公元前 3500 年的老官台、裴李岗、河姆渡、马家浜、仰韶等文化遗址，彰显出先民围绕生存健康问题所做的各种努力。

公元前 4800 年以来，以关中、晋南、豫西为中心形成的仰韶文化，是中原史前文化的重要标志。以半坡、庙底沟类型为典型，自公元前 3500 年走向繁荣，属于锄耕粟黍稻兼营渔猎饲养猪鸡经济方式，彩陶尤其发达。公元前 4400—公元前 3300 年，长江中游的大溪文化，薄胎彩陶和白陶发达。公元前 4300—公元前 2500 年山东丰岛的大汶口文化，红陶为主。公元前 3500 年前后，辽东的红山文化原始宗教发展。公元前 3300 年以来，长江下游由河姆渡、马家浜文化衍续的良渚文化和陇西的马家窑文化、江淮间的薛家岗文化时趋发达。

公元前 2600—公元前 2000 年，黄河中下游龙山文化群形成，冶铸铜器，制作玉器，土坯、石灰、夯筑技术开始应用。公元前 2697 年，轩辕战败炎帝（有说其后裔）、蚩尤而为黄帝纪元元年。黄帝西巡访贤，"至岐见岐伯，引载而归，访于治道"。其引归地"溱洧襟带于前，梅泰环拱于后"，即今河南新密市古城寨。岐黄答问，构建《黄帝内经》健康知识体系，中华文明从关注民生健康起步。颛顼改革宗教，神职人员出现；帝喾修身节用，帝尧和合百国，舜同律度量衡，大禹疏导治水，中华民族不断繁衍昌盛。

公元前 2070 年，禹之子启以豫西晋南为中心建立夏王朝，二里头青铜文化为其特征，半地穴、窑洞、地面建筑并存。饮食卫生器具、酒器增多。朱砂安神作用在宫殿应用。公元前 1600 年，商灭夏。偃师商城设有铸铜作坊。公元前 1300 年，盘庚迁殷，使用甲骨文。武丁时期青铜浑铸、分铸并存。公元前 1056 年，相传周"文王被殷纣拘于羑里，演《周易》，成六十四卦"。公元前 1046 年，武王克商建周，定都镐京。青铜器始铸长篇铭文，周原发掘出微型甲骨文字。公元前 770 年，平王东迁。虢国铸铜柄铁剑。公元前 753 年，秦国设置史官。公元前 707 年出现蝗灾、公元前 613 年出现"哈雷彗星"，均被孔子载入《春秋》。公元前 221 年，秦始皇统一中国，多元一体民族大家庭形成，中华医药卫生文物异彩纷呈。

中国是治史大国，历来重视发展文化博物事业，1955 年成立卫生部中医研究院时就设置医史研究室，1982 年中国医史文献研究所成立时复建中国医史博物馆研究收藏展陈文物。2000—2003 年，经王永炎院士、姚乃礼院长等呼吁，科技部批准立项，由李经纬、梁峻为负责人的团队完成"国家重点医药卫生文物收集调研和保护"项目任务，受到科技部项目验收组专家的高度评价，获中华中医药学会科技进步二等奖。2013 年，在国家出版基金资助下，课题组对部分文物重新拍摄或必要置换、充实民族医药文物后，由西安交通大学出版社编辑、组聘国内一流翻译团队英译说明文字付梓，受到国家中医药博物馆筹备工作领导小组和办公室的高度重视。

"物以类聚"，《图典》主要依据文物质地、种类分为 9 卷，计有陶瓷，金属，纸质，竹木，玉石、织品及标本，壁画石刻及遗址，少数民族文物，其他，备考等卷。同卷下主要根据历史年代或小类分册设章。每卷下的历史时段不求统一。遵循上述规则将《图典》划分为21册，总计收载文物5000余件。对每件文物的描述，除质地、规格、馆藏等基本要素外，重点描述其在民生健康中的作用。对少数暂不明确的事项在括号中注明待考。对引自各博物馆的材料除在文物后列出馆藏外，还在书后再次统一列出馆名或参考书目，以充分尊重其馆藏权，也同时维护本典作者的引用权。

21世纪，围绕人类健康的生命科学将飞速发展，但科学离不开文化，文化离不开文物。发掘文物承载的信息为现实服务，谨引用横渠先生四言之两语："为天地立心，为生民立命"，既作为编撰本《图典》之宗旨，也是我们践行国家"一带一路"倡议的具体努力。希冀通过本《图典》的出版发行，教育国人，提振中华民族精神；走向世界，为人类健康事业贡献力量。

李经纬　梁峻　刘学春

2017年6月于北京

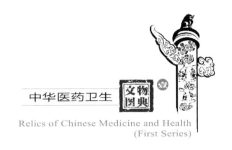

中华医药卫生 文物图典

Relics of Chinese Medicine and Health
(First Series)

目 录

1

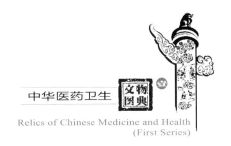

中华医药卫生 文物图典
Relics of Chinese Medicine and Health
(First Series)

Contents

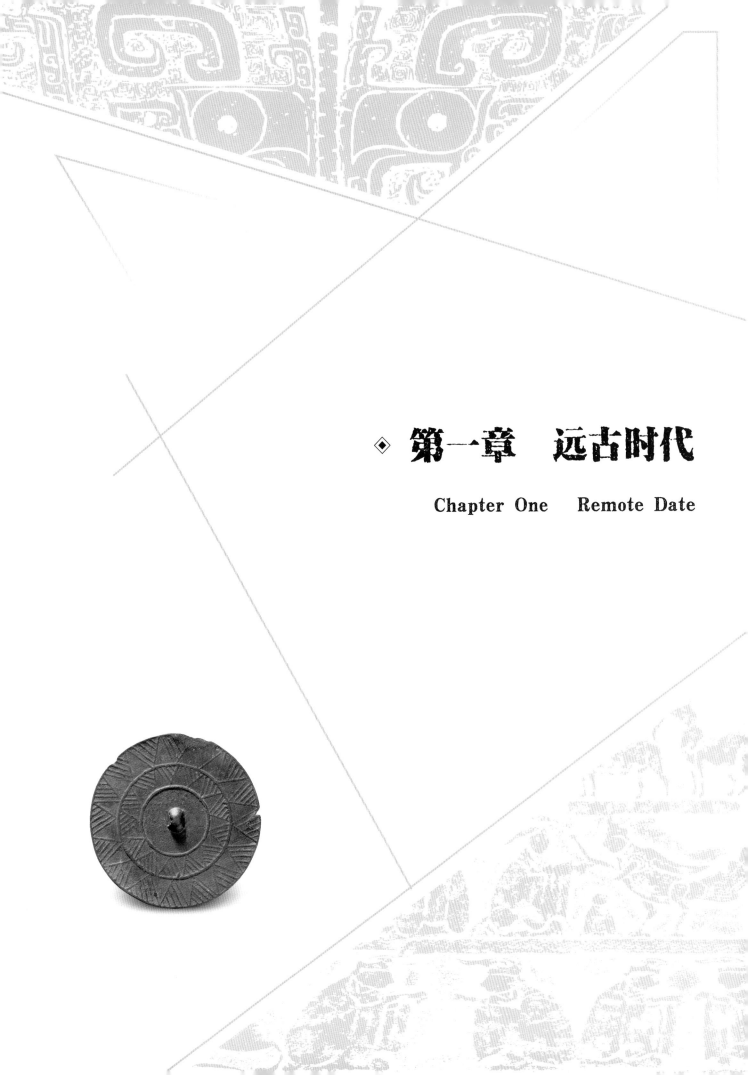

第一章 远古时代

Chapter One　Remote Date

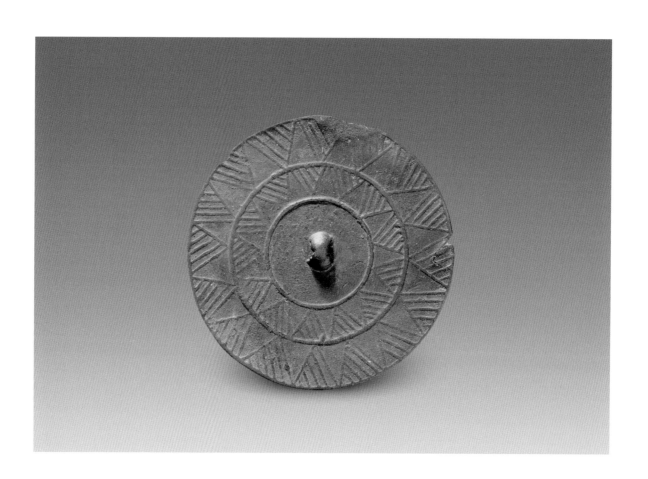

三角纹镜

齐家文化

青铜质

直径 14.6 厘米

Bronze Mirror with Triangle Pattern

Qijia Culture

Bronze

Diameter 14.6 cm

弓形钮，无钮座。钮外饰凸弦纹三周，内圈平
素无纹饰，中圈排列十三组三角纹，角与角间
饰平行斜线，外圈排列十六组三角纹，三角纹
大小不等，不甚规则。此镜纹饰古朴，是我国
目前发现的较早铜镜之一。据传为甘肃省出土。

中国国家博物馆藏

It has an arch-shaped knob with no pedestal.
There are three rings of convex string pattern
around the knob. There is no pattern in the inner
circle. In the middle circle, there are 13 groups of
triangle pattern with parallel oblique lines in the
triangle between every two triangles. In the outer
circle there are 16 groups of triangle pattern of
different sizes. The decoration of the mirror is
simple. It is one of the oldest bronze mirrors that
have been discovered in China. It is said that it
was unearthed in Gansu.

Preserved in National Museum of China

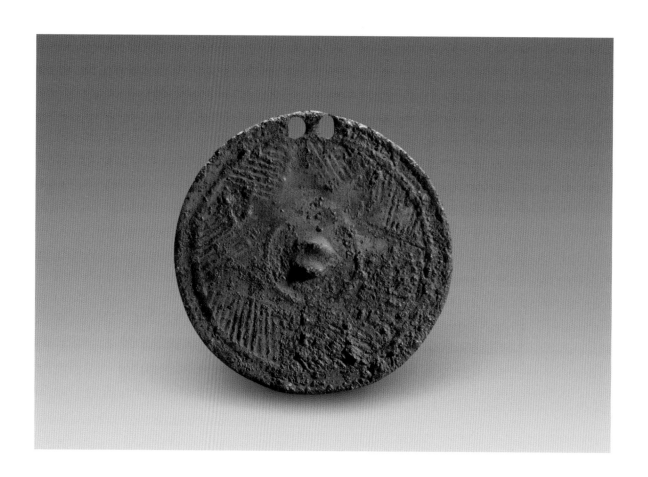

七角纹镜

齐家文化

青铜质

直径 8.9 厘米

Bronze Mirror with Heptangular Pattern

Qijia Culture

Bronze

Diameter 8.9 cm

镜背两弦纹间以三角纹折转成不规则的七角形图案，角与角之间饰斜线纹。镜钮残损，故于边缘处穿两孔，便于系绳悬挂。此镜是中国发现最早的铜镜之一，图案设计精美，铸造工艺高超，具有较高的历史价值和艺术价值。1976 年于青海尕马台出土。

青海省博物馆藏

Within the two-circle pattern on the back of the mirror, there are irregular heptangular motifs made from folded triangular pattern. Between every two triangles is the pattern of oblique lines. Because of the damaged knob, two holes were punched close to the edge of the mirror for tethering and hanging. It is one of the oldest bronze mirrors that have been discovered in China. With exquisite design and superb casting technique, this mirror is of relatively high historical and artistic value. It was unearthed in Gamatai, Qinghai Province.

Preserved in Qinghai Province Museum

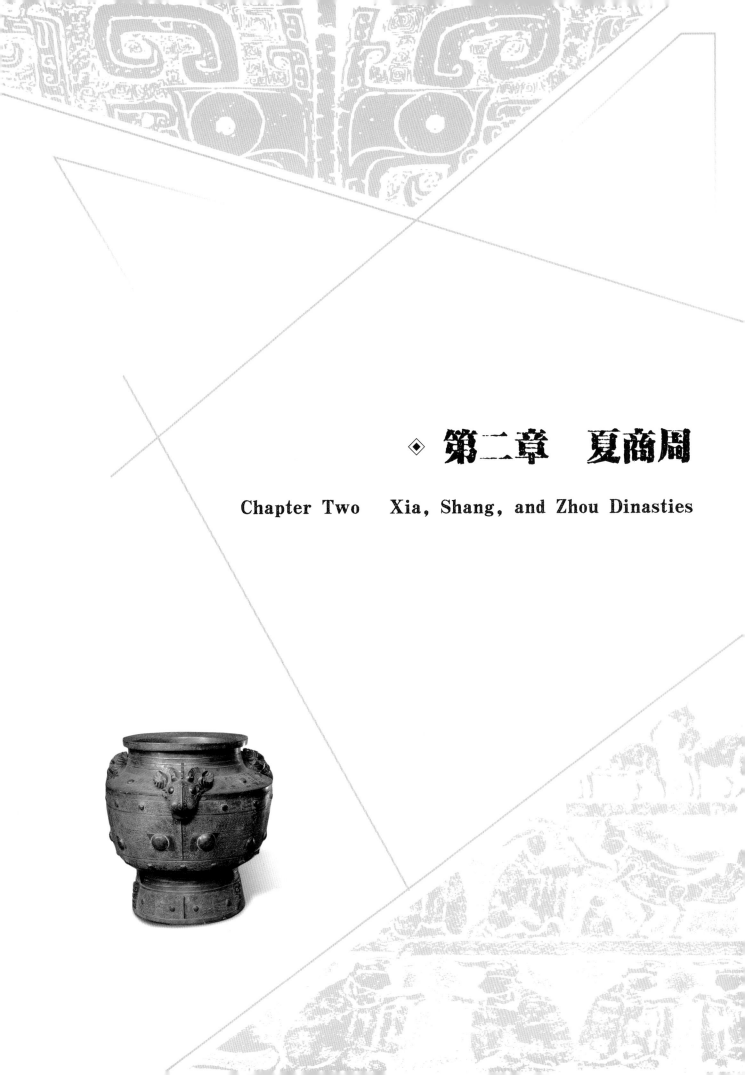

◇ 第二章　夏商周

Chapter Two　Xia, Shang, and Zhou Dinasties

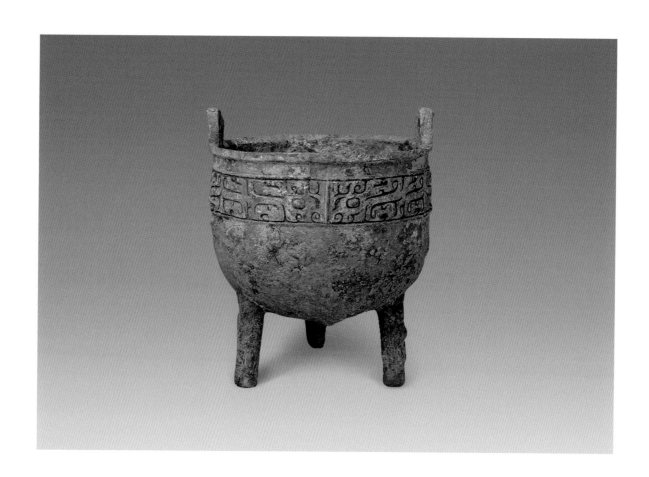

兽面纹鼎

商代早期

青铜质

宽 15.1 厘米，通高 17.1 厘米，重 1.4 千克

Tripod with Animal Mask Pattern

Early Shang Dynasty

Bronze

Width 15.1 cm/ Height 17.1 cm/ Weight 1.4 kg

深圆腹，小耳，柱足矮而细，其中一耳与一
足成直线。口下饰粗线兽面纹。1958 年收购。

故宫博物院藏

The tripod has a deep round belly, small ears,
and short and thin columnar legs. One of the
ears and one of the legs are on a vertical line.
Below the rim of the mouth on the outside,
there is decoration of thick-line animal mask. It
was acquired in 1958.

Preserved in The Palace Museum

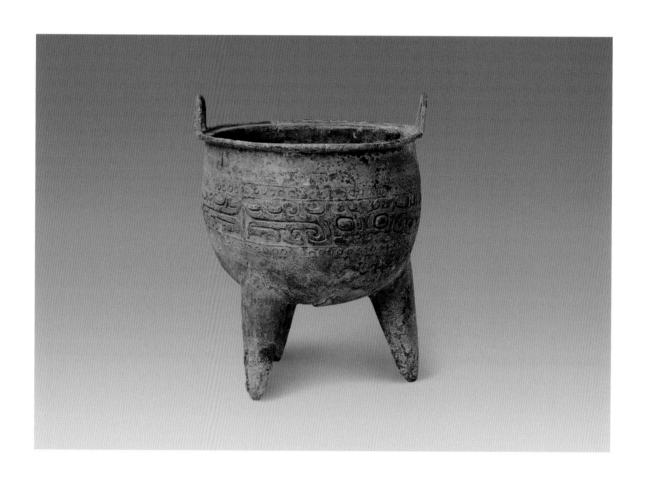

兽面纹鼎

商代早期

青铜质

宽 15.7 厘米，通高 18.9 厘米，重 0.95 千克

Tripod with Animal Mask Pattern

Early Shang Dynasty

Bronze

Width 15.7 cm/ Height 18.9 cm/ Weight 0.95 kg

深腹，有宽折沿，立耳呈圆拱形，口沿下饰
兽面纹带。三个锥形足，中空，一足与一耳
在垂直线上。1957 年收购。

故宫博物院藏

The tripod has a deep belly, a wide folded edge,
and arch-shaped prick ears. Below the rim of the
mouth on the outside, there is decoration of the
design of animal mask. It has hollow tricone-
shaped legs, with one of the legs and one of the
ears on a vertical line. It was acquired in 1957.
Preserved in The Palace Museum

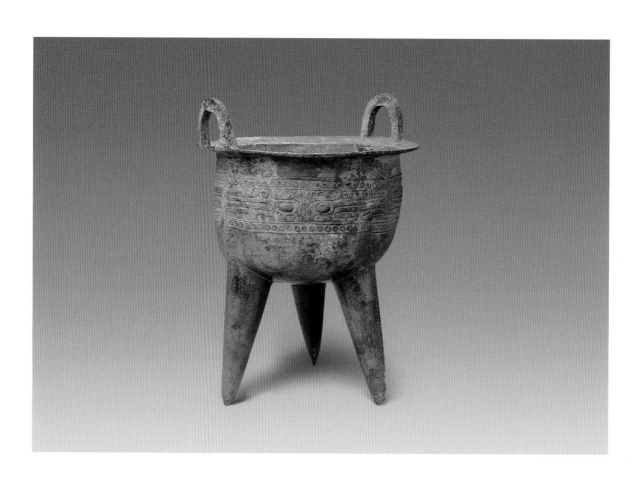

兽面纹鼎

商代早期

青铜质

宽 16.5 厘米，通高 21.1 厘米，重 1.02 千克

Tripod with Animal Mask Pattern

Early Shang Dynasty

Bronze

Width 16.5 cm/ Height 21.1 cm/ Weight 1.02 kg

深腹，小耳，锥形足中空，其中一耳与一足
成直线，形成不平衡状态。口下饰联珠纹镶
边的兽面纹。北京市文化局调拨。

故宫博物院藏

The tripod has a deep belly, small ears, hollow
cone-shaped legs, with one of the ears and one of
the legs on a vertical line, which creates a state
of imbalance of the tripod. Below the rim of the
mouth, there is decoration of the design of animal
mask edged with a pattern of a string of beads on
both sides of the band of animal masks. The tripod
was allocated from Beijing Municipal Bureau of
Culture.

Preserved in The Palace Museum

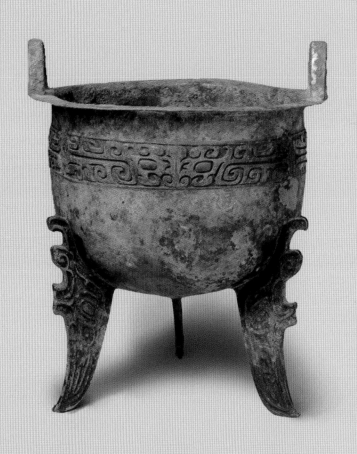

兽面纹鼎

商代早期

青铜质

宽 18.3 厘米，通高 21 厘米，重 1.04 千克

圆体，深腹，平口沿外折，双立耳，三个兽

形扁足呈刀状。颈饰兽面纹，足饰夔纹。

1958 年收购。

故宫博物院藏

Tripod with Animal Mask Pattern

Early Shang Dynasty

Bronze

Width 18.3 cm/ Height 21 cm/ Weight 1.04 kg

The tripod has a round body, a deep belly, a flat
folded edge, and two prick ears. Three animal-
like flat legs are shaped in knives. The neck is
decorated with animal mask pattern and on the
legs are Kui dragon patterns (Kui dragon is a one-
legged monster in fable). It was acquired in 1958.

Preserved in The Palace Museum

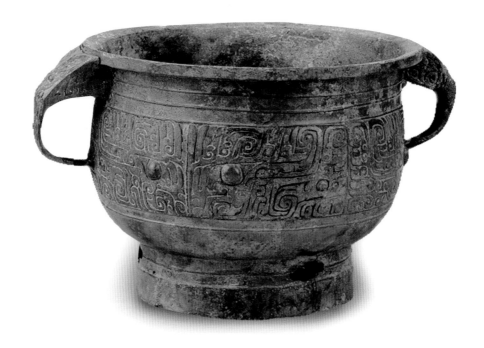

兽面纹簋

商代早期

青铜质

口径 24.5 厘米，通高 17.4 厘米

深圆腹，圈足，平沿外折，二附耳。腹部饰
兽面纹。食器或用于祭祀。

湖北省博物馆藏

Gui with Animal Mask Pattern

Early Shang Dynasty

Bronze

Mouth Diameter 24.5 cm/ Height 17.4 cm

It is a round-mouthed vessel with two loop
handles and ring foot. The belly is decorated with
animal mask patterns, and it was used to contain
cooked food, and it could also served as a
sacrificial vessel.

Preserved in Hubei Provincial Museum

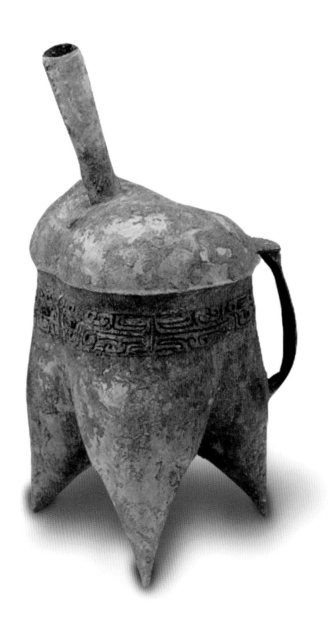

顶流袋足铜盉

商代早期

青铜质

通高 36.4 厘米

顶部有管状冲天流，流两边的乳钉与顶面构成
兽面。袋足中空，腹部饰饕餮纹，侧面为夔纹。
盉盛水以调和酒味浓淡。

湖北省博物馆藏

Bronze He with Top Spout and Bag-like Feet

Early Shang Dynasty

Bronze

Height 36.4 cm

This vessel has a tubular spout that is directed
upwardly, and the nipples on the two sides of the
spout and surface of the top creates an animal
mask pattern. The bag-like structure is hollow
inside, and the belly is decorated with Tao Tie
pattern, and the side surface with Kui dragon
pattern. It was used to keep water to regulate the
taste of wine.

Preserved in Hubei Provincial Museum

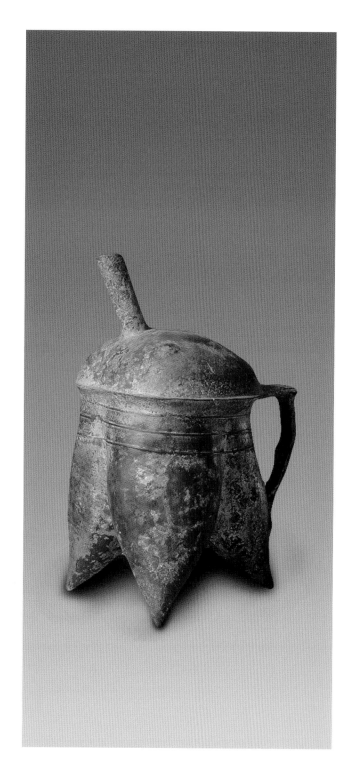

弦纹盉

商代早期

青铜质

宽 14.7 厘米，通高 21.2 厘米，重 1.36 千克

He with Bowstring Pattern

Early Shang Dynasty

Bronze

Width 14.7 cm/ Height 21.2 cm/ Weight 1.36 kg

上部为半圆，下部有三袋状尖足。前有一管状流，后

面有一桃形口，颈部有一圈窄沿外凸，下饰弦纹。

1956 年文化部文物管理局调拨。

故宫博物院藏

The upper part of the vessel is half round in shape and

the lower part is formed into a shape of three bag-like

sharp legs. On its forepart, there is a tubular spout. On

its back, there is a peach-shaped mouth. On the neck,

there is a circle of fine protruding edge, with bowstring

patterns below. It was allocated from Cultural Relics

Administration of the Ministry of Culture.

Preserved in The Palace Museum

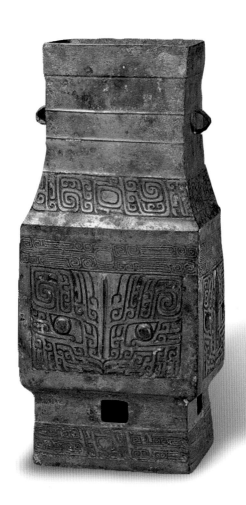

兽面纹方壶

商代早期

青铜质

口径 10.4 厘米 ×7.3 厘米，宽 13.8 厘米，高 28.1 厘米，
重 1.38 千克

壶体呈扁方形，双耳，长方圈足，足上有四个穿孔。颈部饰
弦纹二道，肩、足各饰一圈目雷纹，腹饰兽面纹。1959 年
北京市文化局调拨。

故宫博物院藏

Square Bronze Pot with Animal Mask Pattern

Early Shang Dynasty

Bronze

Mouth Diameter 10.4 cm×7.3 cm/ Width 13.8 cm/ Height 28.1 cm/
Weight 1.38 kg

The jar has a flattened square shape, a pair of ears, and a long
and a square ring foot with four perforations on it. The neck
is decorated with two belts of bowstring patterns. The vessel
shoulder and foot are respectively decorated with a circle of
eye-like designs and thunder pattern. The belly is decorated
with beast face mask. It was allocated from Beijing Municipal
Bureau of Culture in 1959.

Preserved in The Palace Museum

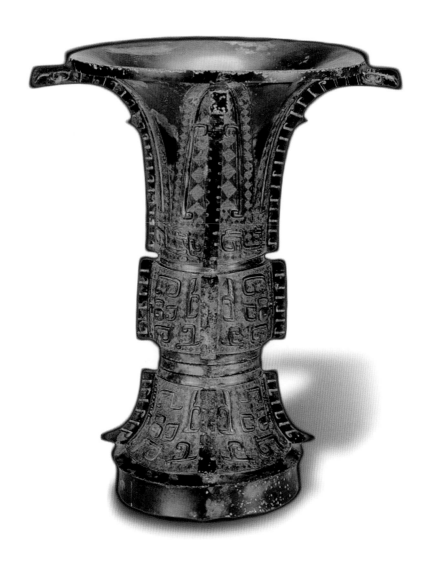

天兽御尊

商代早期

青铜质

口径 26.4 厘米，通高 37.1 厘米

酒器，敞口，器身饰满花纹，云雷纹衬底，颈饰蕉叶纹，其下饰回首夔纹，器身从上至下起四条侈口沿的扉棱。圈足内铸铭文"天兽御"。1965 年湖北省武汉市汉南区纱帽山出土。

湖北省博物馆藏

Zun with Characters "Tian Shou Yu"

Early Shang Dynasty

Bronze

Mouth Diameter 26.4 cm/ Height 37.1 cm

This is a wine vessel with a flared mouth. Its body is decorated with flower pattern with cloud and thunder pattern as the ground-tint. Its neck is decorated with the pattern of banana leaf. The lower part of the vessel is decorated with the pattern of Kui dragon that looks back. From top to bottom of the vessel there are four strip ridges around which run beyond the mouth rim. On the ring foot, there is an inscription of three characters "Tian Yu Shou". It was unearthed in Hannan District of Wuhan, Hubei Province

Preserved in Hubei Provincial Museum

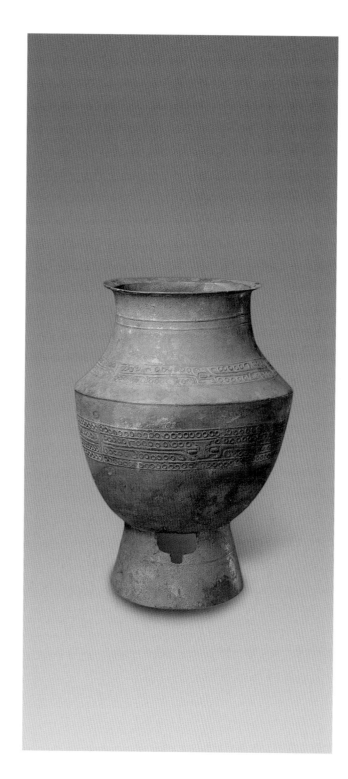

兽面纹尊

商代早期

青铜质

宽 24.1 厘米，通高 32.4 厘米，重 3.03 千克

Zun with Animal Mask Pattern

Early Shang Dynasty

Bronze

Width 24.1 cm/ Height 32.4 cm/ Weight 3.03 kg

直口，卷沿，高颈，宽肩，鼓腹，圈足。颈、足均饰弦纹，肩饰联珠纹镶边目纹，腹部饰兽面纹和联珠纹，圈足上有十字镂孔。1958 年收购。

故宫博物院藏

The vessel has a straight mouth with curled rims, a long neck, a broad shoulder, a swelling belly, and a ring foot. The neck and foot are decorated with bowstring pattern and the shoulder is decorated with eye-like pattern with square thunder pattern edged with design of a circle of a string of beads. The belly is decorated with design of beast face and pattern of a string of beads. There is a cross hollowed-out hole on the ring foot. The relic was acquired in 1958.

Preserved in The Palace Museum

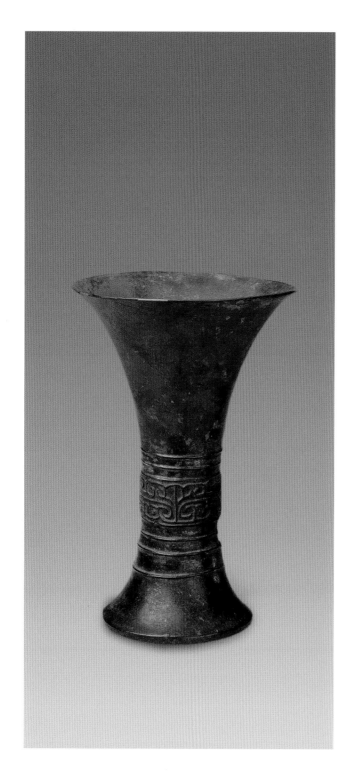

兽面纹觚

商代早期

青铜质

通高 15.1 厘米，宽 10.7 厘米，重 0.37 千克

Gu with Animal Mask Pattern

Early Shang Dynasty

Bronze

Height 15.1 cm/ Width 10.7 cm/ Weight 0.37 kg

敞口，束腰，圈足。器身细长。腰饰兽面纹
和弦纹。清宫旧藏。

故宫博物院藏

The vessel has an open mouth, a slender waist,
and a ring foot. The body is tall and slender.
There is beast face pattern and a bowstring
pattern in the middle of the vessel. It was an
antique from the imperial palace of the Qing
Dynasty.

Preserved in The Palace Museum

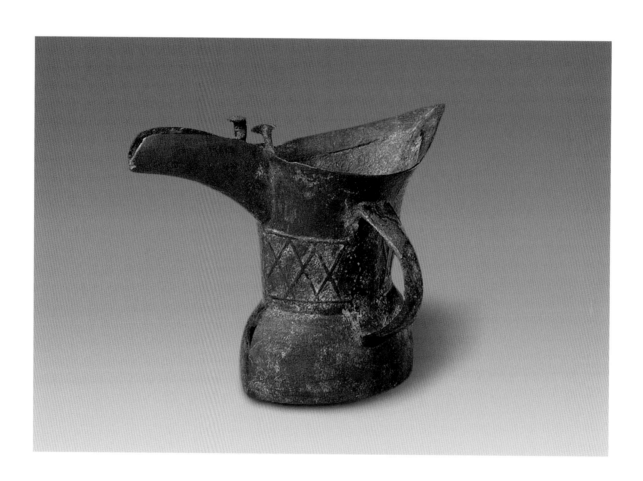

网纹爵

商代早期

青铜质

宽 14.1 厘米，通高 9.2 厘米，重 0.22 千克

Jue with Reticulate Pattern

Early Shang Dynasty

Bronze

Width 14.1 cm/ Height 9.2 cm/ Weight 0.22 kg

敞口，窄流，尖尾，钉状柱，束腰，腹外侈，

腰腹间有明显分界，平底。腰饰网纹。三足残。

1959 年收购。

故宫博物院藏

The vessel is openmouthed, with a narrow
spout, a sharp tail, and two nail-shaped pillars
on the mouth. The vessel has a wasp waist.
The belly slightly tilts outward, and there is a
clear dividing line between the waist and the
belly. The vessel has a flat bottom. The waist
is decorated with a netlike design. Its three feet
are not intact. It was acquired in 1959.

Preserved in The Palace Museum

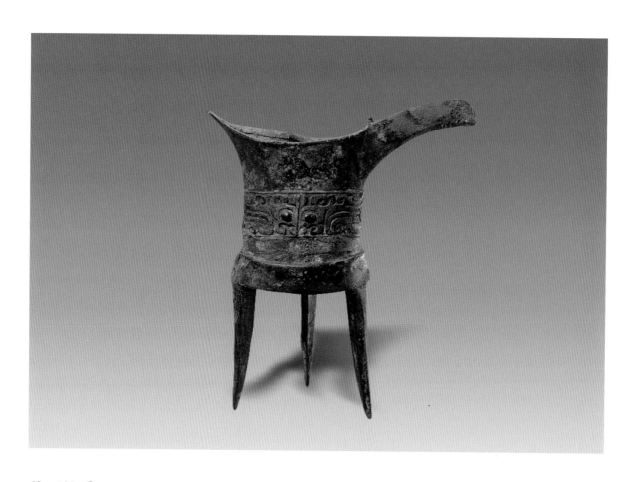

兽面纹爵

商代早期

青铜质

宽 14.8 厘米，通高 16.1 厘米，重 0.24 千克

Jue with Animal Mask Pattern

Early Shang Dynasty

Bronze

Width 14.8 cm/ Height 16.1 cm/ Weight 0.24 kg

椭圆形口，窄长流，短尾，薄壁，矮柱立于流口，束腰，平底，三棱锥足略向外侈。腹饰兽面纹。1956 年收购。

故宫博物院藏

The vessel has an oval mouth with a long narrow spout, a short tail, and thin walls. There is a short pillar in the mouth of the spout. The vessel has a wasp waist, a flat bottom, and a triangular pyramid foot that slightly tilts outward. The belly is decorated with beast face pattern. It was acquired in 1956.

Preserved in The Palace Museum

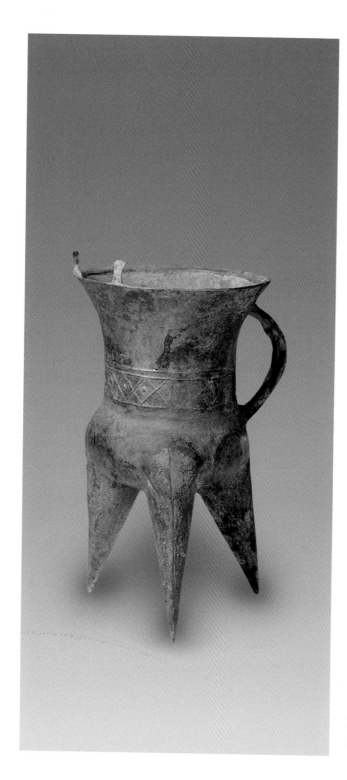

网纹斝

商代早期

青铜质

宽 17.1 厘米，通高 25.8 厘米，重 0.93 千克

Jia with Reticulate Pattern

Early Shang Dynasty

Bronze

Width 17.1 cm/ Height 25.8 cm/ Weight 0.93 kg

圆体，侈口，口上有二小柱，腹上有一素錾，
腹下有三锥状足，足中空。腹部饰网纹。
1957 年收购。

故宫博物院藏

This round vessel has a large flared mouth on
which there are two small columns. There is a
simple handle on the belly, and there are hollow
tripodal taper feet. The belly is decorated with
net like pattern. This vessel was acquired in
1957.

Preserved in The Palace Museum

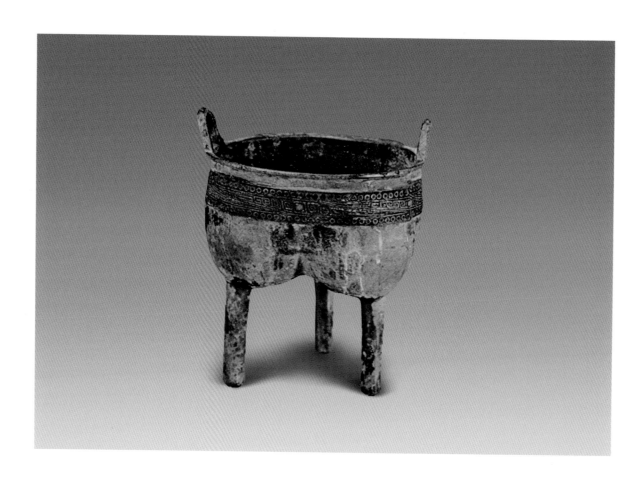

雷纹分裆鼎

商代晚期

青铜质

口径 16.6 厘米，通高 20 厘米

Separated Crotch Tripod with Thunder Pattern

Late Shang Dynasty

Bronze

Mouth Diameter 16.6 cm/ Height 20 cm

立耳，直口狭唇，高腹较浅，分裆线近鼎口，下承三柱足。腹上部饰一周斜角雷纹带，联珠纹框于雷纹带上下。

山西博物院藏

The tripod has prick ears, a straight and narrow lip, and a high but shallow belly with the open crotch line close to the top and meeting with three columnar legs under the belly. There is a band of oblique-line square pattern around the upper part of belly. A line of the pattern of a string of beads edges the band on both sides.

Preserved in Shanxi Museum

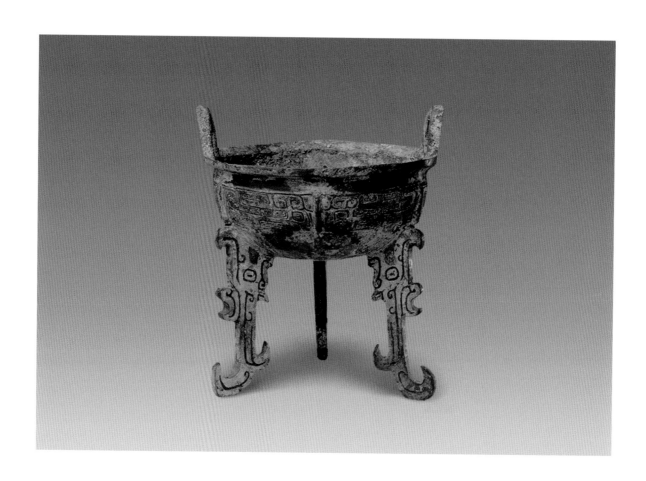

☒ 鼎

商代晚期

青铜质

宽 14.5 厘米，通高 15.8 厘米，重 0.76 千克

Tripod with Character "☒"

Late Shang Dynasty

Bronze

Width 14.5 cm/ Height 15.8 cm/ Weight 0.76 kg

体圆，腹呈半球形，双立耳，三扁足。足呈夔
形张嘴托住器腹，夔尾上卷呈钩状，腹上有六
凸棱，以凸棱为鼻，饰兽面纹三。铭文"▨"
字在器内底。传河南安阳出土，1960 年北京市
文化局调拨。

故宫博物院藏

The tripod is round in shape, with a hemisphere-
like belly, two prick ears, and three flat legs.
The legs are in the shape of a "Kui", a one-
legged mythical animal in fable and opening its
mouth to hold up the belly and its tail rolling
up shaped like a hook. There are six ridges on
the belly that serve as Kui's nose, and animal
masks are cast. The inscription of ▨ is on the
bottom. It is said that the tripod was unearthed
in Anyang, Henan Province. The tripod was
allocated from Beijing Municipal Bureau of
Culture in 1960.

Preserved in The Palace Museum

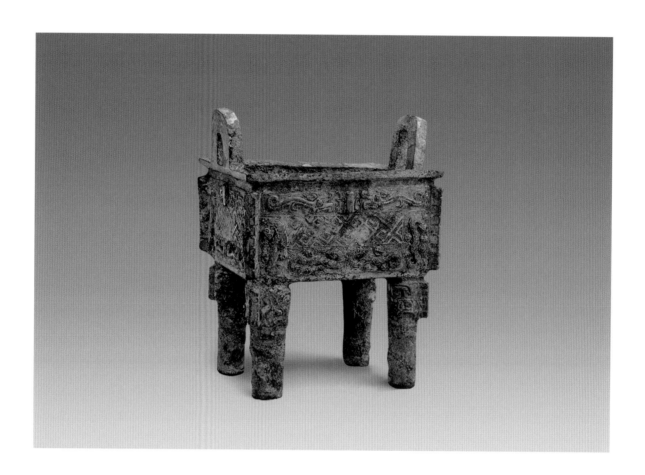

▨方鼎

商代晚期

青铜质

口长 18.3 厘米，口宽 14.2 厘米，通高 23.7 厘米，重 3.04 千克

Quadripod Caldron with Character "▨"

Late Shang Dynasty

Bronze

Mouth Length 18.3 cm/ Mouth Width 14.2 cm/ Height 23.7 cm/ Weight 3.04 kg

长方体，直壁，深腹，平底，口沿外折，口上有双立耳，腹下四柱足。腹部四角、颈部及足上均有凸棱，颈饰夔纹。腹中部饰勾连雷纹，左、右、下三方饰蛇纹，足饰兽面纹。铭文一"▨"字在器内壁上。1946 年入藏。

故宫博物院藏

The quadripod is a cuboid with straight walls, a deep belly, a flat bottom, a mouth with folded edge, two prick ears on the mouth, and four columnar legs under the belly. There are ridges on each of the belly's four corners, the neck, and the legs. The neck is decorated with the Kui dragon pattern. In the central part of the belly, there is connected thunder pattern. The left, right and lower parts of the belly are decorated with the design of snakes, and there is the design of animal mask on the legs. There is an inscription of ▨ on the inner wall of the quadripod. It was collected in 1946.

Preserved in The Palace Museum

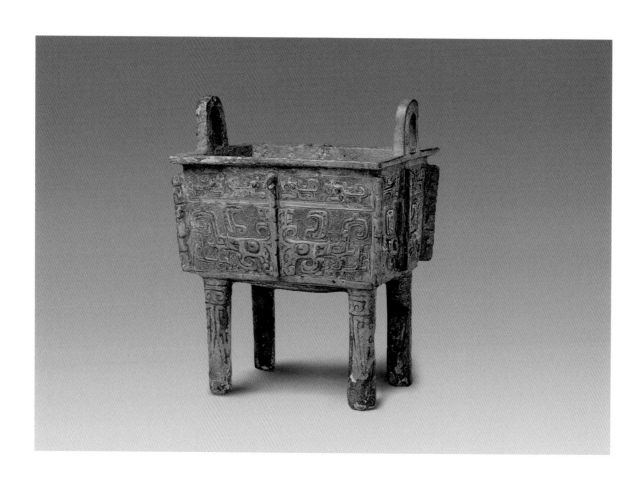

亚酰父已方鼎

商代晚期

青铜质

宽 18.3 厘米，通高 22.7 厘米，重 2.6 千克

Quadripod Caldron with Characters Including "酰"

Late Shang Dynasty

Bronze

Width 18.3 cm/ Height 22.7 cm/ Weight 2.6 kg

长方体，深腹，平底，口沿外折，双立耳，
四柱足。颈部和腹四角均有凸棱，颈饰鸟纹
一圈，腹饰兽面纹，足根部饰云雷纹一圈，
下有三垂叶纹。铭文"亚醜父己"2 行 4 字
在器内。1954 年国家文物局调拨。

故宫博物院藏

The quadripod is a cuboid with a deep belly, a flat bottom, a mouth with folded edge, two prick ears, and four columnar legs. There are ridges on the neck and the four corners of the belly. The neck is decorated with a ring of bird pattern, while the belly is decorated with animal-mask designs. At the heels of the feet, there is a ring of cloud-and-thunder designs with the pattern of three hanging leaves. There is an inscription of 4 characters in 2 lines inside the quadripod. The quadripod was allocated from State Administration of Cultural Heritage in 1954.

Preserved in The Palace Museum

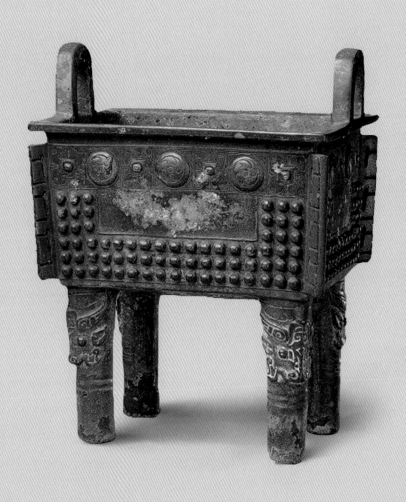

亚酰父丁方鼎

商代晚期

青铜质

宽 18.3 厘米，通高 22.7 厘米，重 3.12 千克

长方体，深腹，平底，口沿外折，双立耳，四柱足。腹四角有凸棱，颈饰四瓣花纹，间饰圆涡纹，腹部饰乳丁三行呈凹形排列，中间部分光素无纹。足根部饰兽面纹，下有弦纹一道。铭文"亚酰父丁"1 行 4 字在器内壁上。1956 年北京市文化局调拨。

故宫博物院藏

Quadripod Caldron with Characters Including "酰"

Late Shang Dynasty

Bronze

Width 18.3 cm/ Height 22.7 cm/ Weight 3.12 kg

The quadripod is a cuboid with a deep belly, a flat bottom, a mouth with folded edge, two prick ears, and four columnar legs. There is a ridge on each of the four corners of the belly. The neck is decorated with the design of a flower of four petals with vortex pattern embedded among them. Three lines of nipple pattern are arranged on the belly in a concave shape, the central part of which is free of designs. The heels are decorated with animal-mask designs and there is a raised line design in its lower part. There is a 4-character inscription in one line on the inner wall of the quadripod. The guadripod was allocated from Beijing Municipal Bureau of Culture in 1956.

Preserved in The Palace Museum

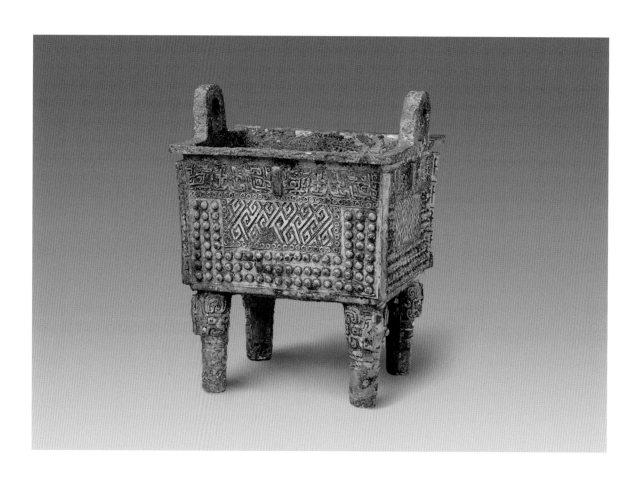

羊父丁方鼎

商代晚期

青铜质

宽 17.1 厘米，通高 21.3 厘米，重 3.12 千克

Quadripod Caldron with Characters "Yang Fu Ding"

Late Shang Dynasty

Bronze

Width 17.1 cm/ Height 21.3 cm/ Weight 3.12 kg

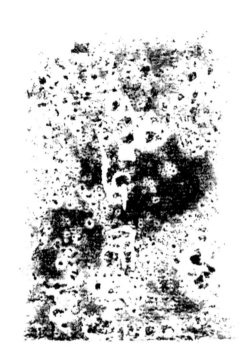

长方体，直壁，深腹，平底，口沿外折，口上有双立耳，腹下有四柱足。腹部四角、颈部、足上均有凸棱，腹中部饰勾连雷纹，左、右及下方各饰三道乳丁纹。颈和足饰兽面纹。铭文1行4字在器内壁上。1956年收购。

故宫博物院藏

The caldron is a cuboid with straight vertical walls, a deep belly, a flat bottom, a mouth with folded edge, two prick ears, and four columnar legs under the belly. There is a ridge on the neck, each of the legs, and each of the four corners of the belly. There is connected thunder-pattern decoration on the central part of the belly, while the left, the right and the lower parts of the belly are decorated with three lines of nipple designs. The neck and the legs are decorated with animal-mask designs. There is inscription of 4 characters in one line on the inner wall of the caldron. The caldron was acquired in 1956.

Preserved in The Palace Museum

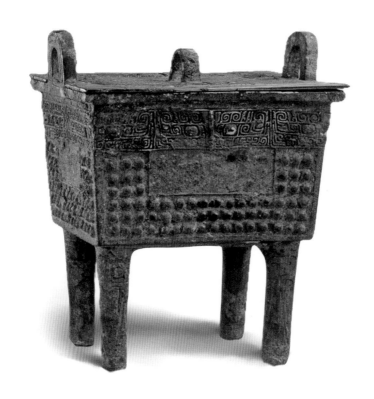

田告方鼎

商代晚期

青铜质

宽 15 厘米，通高 15.6 厘米，重 1.68 千克

Quadripod Caldron with Characters "Tian Gao"

Late Shang Dynasty

Bronze

Width 15 cm/ Height 15.6 cm/ Weight 1.68 kg

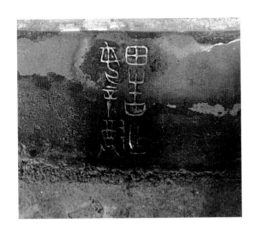

长方形器体，四柱足，口沿二直耳。有盖，盖上有一半圆形钮。器四面的颈上均饰兽面纹。腹部中心为素面，左、右两侧和下部均饰乳丁纹三行。足上饰三角云纹。盖与器对铭，各有铭文 2 行 6 字，记田告为其母辛做祭器。陕西宝鸡出土，1956 年冯公度先生家属捐献。

故宫博物院藏

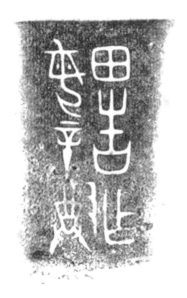

The quadripod caldron is a cuboid with four columnar legs, and two prick ears. It has a cover, on which there is a semicircle-shaped knob. The neck on the four sides of the quadripod is decorated with animal-mask designs. There is no decoration on the central part of the belly. The left, the right, and the lower parts of the belly are decorated with three lines of nipple designs. There are triangular cloud designs on the legs. There is a pair of inscriptions on the cover and the quadripod caldron respectively, which are six characters in two lines each, meaning that this quadripod was dedicated by Tian Gao as a sacrificial utensil for his mother. It was unearthed in Baoji, Shaanxi Province, and donated to the museum by Mr. Feng Gongdu's family in 1956.

Preserved in The Palace Museum

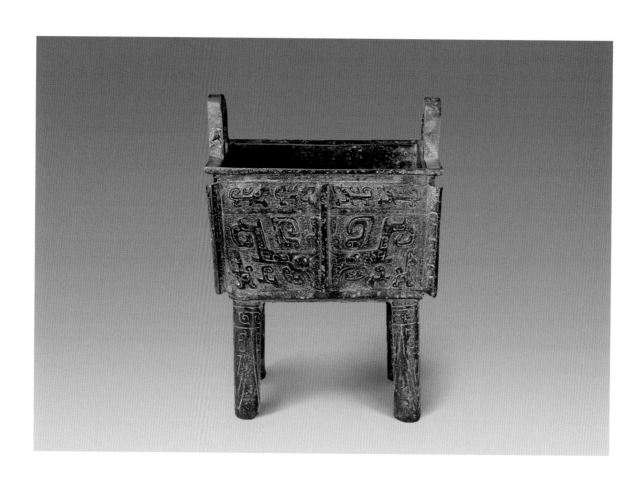

小臣 方鼎

商代晚期

青铜质

口长 22.5 厘米，通高 29.6 厘米，重 6.18 千克

Quadripod Caldron with Characters Including " "

Late Shang Dynasty

Bronze

Mouth Length 22.5 cm/ Height 29.6 cm/ Weight 6.18 kg

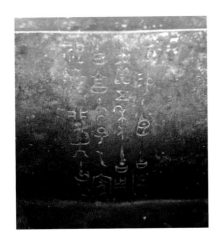

鼎身呈长方形，折沿，双立耳，四柱足。器壁四角及正中均起棱脊，口沿下饰夔纹，腹饰兽面纹，以细密的雷纹为衬地，夔纹和兽面纹上再饰以流畅的线刻。双耳外侧饰线刻云雷纹，足饰线刻云纹及蕉叶纹。方鼎内壁有铭文 4 行 22 字。清宫旧物（原藏颐和园）。

故宫博物院藏

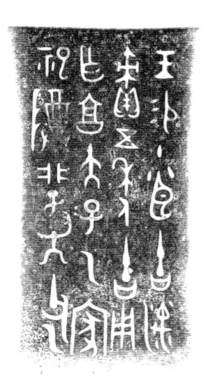

The quadripod is a cuboid with folded edges, two prick ears, and four columnar legs. There is a vertical ridge in the middle of the body and on each of the four corners of the vessel walls. Below the rim of the mouth on the outside, there are designs of "Kui", a legendary monster, while the belly is decorated with animal-mask designs with fine thunder pattern in the background. On the Kui drangon pattern and the animal mask designs, there are decorations of fine smooth flowing lines. The outer side of the ears is decorated with line-form cloud and thunder pattern, while the legs are engraved with line form cloud pattern and banana leaf designs. There is inscription of 22 characters in 4 lines engraved on the inner wall of the vessel. It is an antique from the imperial palace of the Qing Dynasty (originally collected by the Summer Palace).
Preserved in The Palace Museum

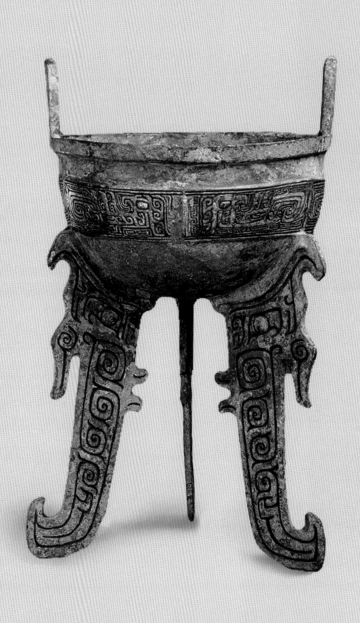

正鼎

商代晚期

青铜质

宽 21.8 厘米，通高 35.5 厘米，重 4.36 千克

圆体，浅腹，双立耳，三扁足呈夔形，夔张嘴托住器腹，夔尾上卷呈钩状。腹饰夔纹，足饰目纹及云雷纹。铭文"正"字在器内底。1946 年入藏。

故宫博物院藏

Tripod with Character "Zheng"

Late Shang Dynasty

Bronze

Width 21.8 cm/ Height 35.5 cm/ Weight 4.36 kg

The tripod is round in shape with a shallow belly, two prick ears, and three flat legs in the shape of "Kui", a legendary monster, with its mouth opening up to hold up the belly and the tail rolling up like a hook. The belly is decorated with Kui dragon pattern, while the legs are decorated with patterns of eyes and cloud and thunder design. The inscription of the character "Zheng" is on the bottom inside the tripod. It was collected in 1946.

Preserved in The Palace Museum

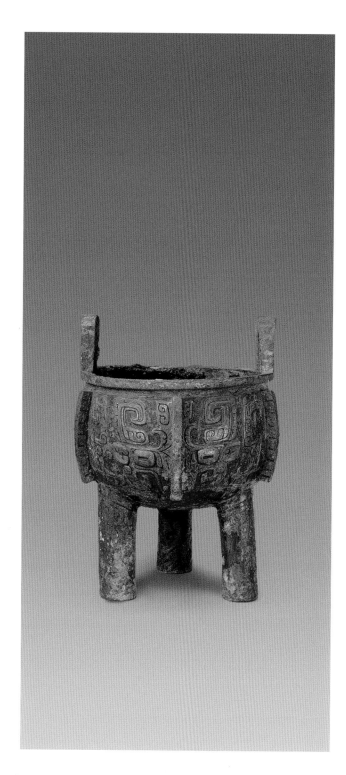

作父乙鼎

商代晚期

青铜质

宽 24 厘米，通高 28.7 厘米，重 6.88 千克

Tripod with Characters "Zuo Fu Yi"

Late Shang Dynasty

Bronze

Width 24 cm/ Height 28.7 cm/ Weight 6.88 kg

圆体，深腹，双立耳，三柱足。腹有六凸棱，以凸棱为鼻组成三组兽面纹，足饰蕉叶纹。内腹铸铭文 2 行 5 字。河南安阳出土，1954 年收购。

故宫博物院藏

The tripod is round in shape with a deep belly, two prick ears, and three columnar legs. On the belly, there are six ridges, and there are three animal mask designs with a ridge as the nose. The legs are decorated with banana leaf pattern. The inscription of 5 characters in 2 lines is on the inner inside of the belly. It was unearthed in Anyang, Henan Province, and acquired in 1954. Preserved in The Palace Museum

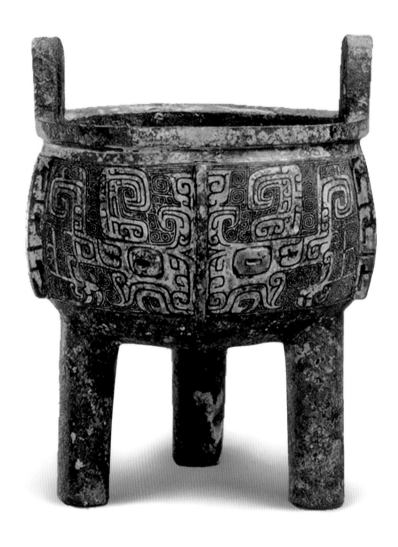

无终鼎

商代晚期

青铜质

宽 16 厘米，通高 21 厘米，重 2.7 千克

圆体，深腹，双立耳，三柱足。腹部有六凸棱，以凸棱为鼻，饰兽面纹。器内壁铸有方国名"无终"，此国名是裘锡圭先生考释的。1957 年收购。

故宫博物院藏

Tripod with Characters "Wu Zhong"

Late Shang Dynasty

Bronze

Width 16 cm/ Height 21 cm/ Weight 2.7 kg

The tripod is round in shape with a deep belly, two prick ears, and three columnar legs. On the belly, there are six ridges designed as noses to form the pattern of animal masks. On the inner wall of the tripod is the inscription of characters "Wu Zhong", a name of a country, which was confirmed by Mr. Qiu Xigui through his investigative studies. It was acquired in 1957.

Preserved in The Palace Museum

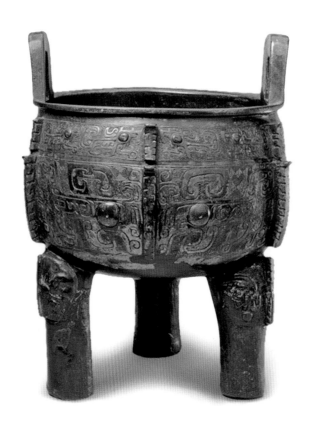

屮 鼎

商代晚期

青铜质

宽 51 厘米，通高 35.3 厘米，重 9.74 千克

Tripod with Character "屮"

Late Shang Dynasty

Bronze

Width 51 cm/ Height 35.3 cm/ Weight 9.74 kg

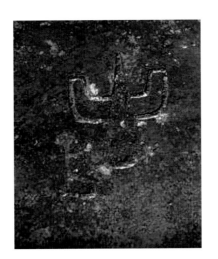 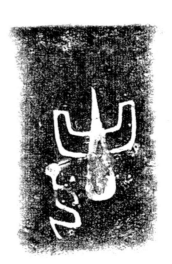

圆体，大腹，三足，双立耳。颈及腹各饰六凸棱，颈饰夔纹，腹饰大兽面纹。足上各有一凸棱，以棱为鼻饰兽面纹。器内壁上有族铭"　"。清宫旧藏。

故宫博物院藏

The tripod is round in shape with a huge belly, three legs, and two prick ears. There are six ridges on the neck and the belly, respectively. The neck is decorated with the designs of "Kui", a legendary monster, and the belly with big animal-mask designs. On each leg, there is one ridge that serves as a nose to form the designs of an animal-mask. An inscription of the family name "　" is on the inner wall of the vessel. It is an antique from the imperial palace of the Qing Dynasty.

Preserved in The Palace Museum

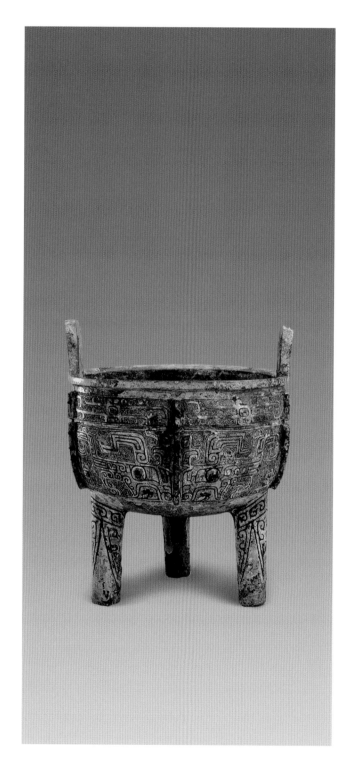

戓鼎

商代晚期

青铜质

宽 18.7 厘米，通高 21.4 厘米，重 2.08 千克

Tripod with Character "戓"

Late Shang Dynasty

Bronze

Width 18.7 cm/ Height 21.4 cm/ Weight 2.08 kg

圆体，深腹，双立耳，三柱足。颈及腹各有
六凸棱，颈饰目纹，腹饰大兽面纹，足饰蕉
叶纹。器内壁有铭文"或"字。1946 年入藏。

故宫博物院藏

The tripod is round in shape with a deep
belly, two prick ears, and three columnar legs.
There are six ridges on the neck and the belly,
respectively. The neck is decorated with eye
designs, and the belly is decorated with designs
of big animal masks, and the legs with banana
leaf designs. The inscription of character "或" is
on the inner wall of the tripod. It was collected
in 1946.

Preserved in The Palace Museum

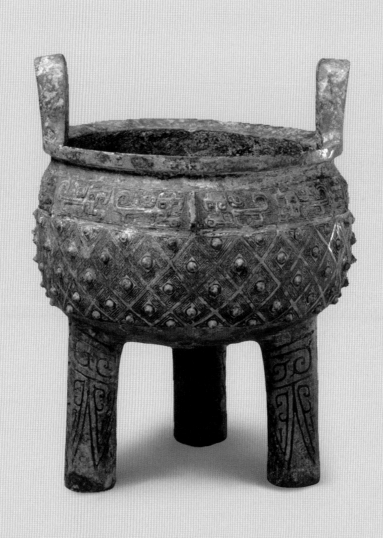

尹鼎

商代晚期

青铜质

宽 16.6 厘米，通高 24.4 厘米，重 2.5 千克

圆体，鼓腹，双立耳，三柱足。颈部饰六凸棱

间饰夔纹，腹饰菱形云雷纹及乳丁，足饰蕉叶纹。

器内壁有一"尹"字。1957 年收购。

故宫博物院藏

Tripod with Character "Yi"

Late Shang Dynasty

Bronze

Width 16.6 cm/ Height 24.4 cm/ Weight 2.5 kg

The tripod is round in shape with a bulged belly,
two prick ears, and three columnar legs. There
are six ridges on the neck, among which there
are designs of "Kui", a monster in fable. The
belly is decorated with diamond-form (cloud and
thunder) design and nipple pattern, and the legs
are decorated with banana leaf designs. There is a
character "Yi" on the inner wall of the tripod. It
was acquired in 1957.

Preserved in The Palace Museum

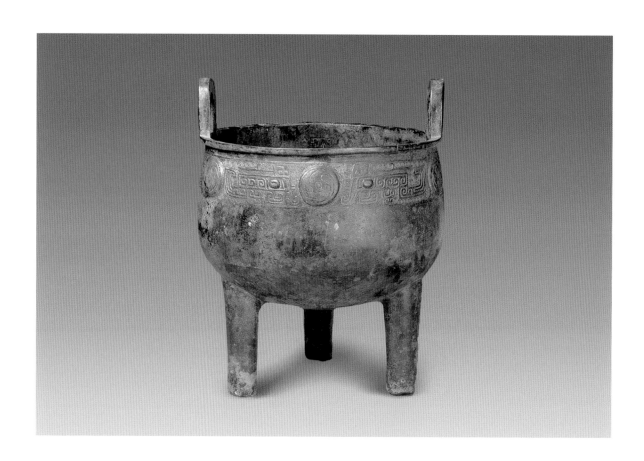

历祖己鼎

商代晚期

青铜质

宽 28.9 厘米，通高 35 厘米，重 8.7 千克

Tripod with Characters "Li Zu Ji"

Late Shang Dynasty

Bronze

Width 28.9 cm/ Height 35 cm/ Weight 8.7 kg

圆体，硕腹，双立耳，三柱足。颈饰夔纹，间饰涡纹。器内壁有铭文 2 行 7 字，记历为祖父己做彝器。亚俞是历家族的族名。清宫旧藏。

故宫博物院藏

The tripod is round in shape with a big belly, two prick ears, and three columnar legs. The neck is decorated with Kui dragon pattern, a monster in fable, with vortex pattern in it. There is an inscription of 7 characters in 2 lines on the inner wall of the tripod, meaning that the tripod was made by a man named "Li" for his grandfather. The characters "Ya Yu" refers to the family name of Li's family. It is an antique from the heritage of the imperial palace of the Qing Dynasty.

Preserved in The Palace Museum

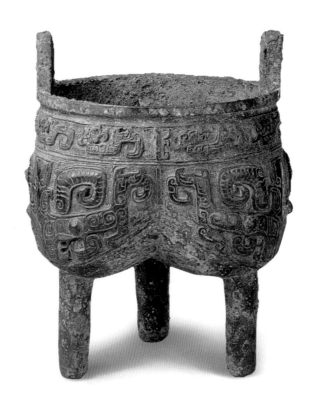

旋鼎

商代晚期

青铜质

宽 18 厘米，通高 22.5 厘米，重 2.9 千克

Tripod with Character "旋"

Late Shang Dynasty

Bronze

Width 18 cm/ Height 22.5 cm/ Weight 2.9 kg

圆体，深腹，双立耳，三柱足。腹饰三兽面，兽面采用浮雕手法，使兽面凸起，周围用雷纹衬托。口下饰虺纹一圈。器内底有族名"旋"字。1946 年入藏。

故宫博物院藏

The tripod is round in shape with a deep belly, two prick ears, and three columnar legs. The belly is decorated with designs of three animal masks. The designs of animal masks reveal the use of the relief technique, so the animal faces are raised from the surface to make the faces raised, and thunder pattern is used as the background. Under the mouth is a ring of snake pattern. There is a character "旋", the family name, on the bottom inside the tripod. It was collected in 1946.

Preserved in The Palace Museum

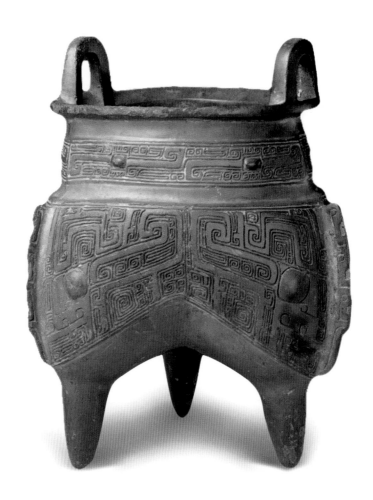

兽面纹鼎

商代晚期

青铜质

宽 17.8 厘米，通高 23 厘米，重 1.97 千克

口有侈唇，有窄直缘，上立双厚耳，颈呈不规则的收束，腹似鬲而宽，下具三个锥形长足。颈饰夔纹，腹饰兽面纹。安徽省阜南县出土。

故宫博物院藏

Tripod with Animal Mask Pattern

Late Shang Dynasty

Bronze

Width 17.8 cm/ Height 23 cm/ Weight 1.97 kg

The tripod has a thick lip on the mouth, narrow and vertical edge, on which stand two fat ears. The neck collects in an irregular shape and the belly is like that of Li, an ancient cooking tripod with hollow legs, but wider, and below the belly there are three cone-shaped long legs. The neck is decorated with designs of "Kui", a legendary monster, and the belly has animal mask pattern. It was unearthed in Funan County, Anhui Province.

Preserved in The Palace Museum

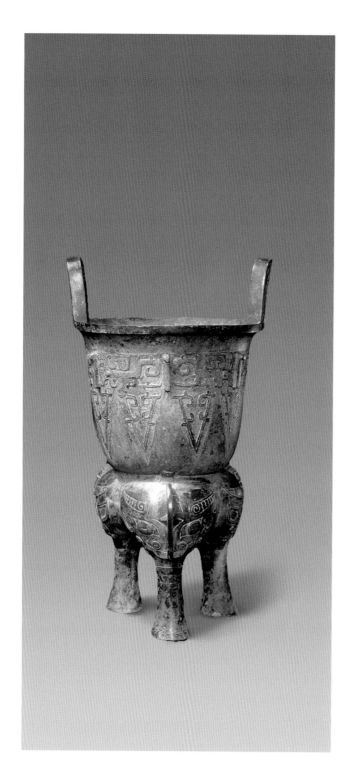

兽面纹甗

商代晚期

青铜质

口径 44.9 厘米，高 80.9 厘米，重 40.02 千克

Yan with Animal Mask Pattern

Late Shang Dynasty

Bronze

Mouth Diameter 44.9 cm/ Height 80.9 cm/

Weight 40.02 kg

由甑、鬲两部分连接而成，腰间有箅。侈口，双立耳，三蹄形足。腹部纹饰以细密的雷纹为地，上部饰兽面纹，下饰蕉叶形夔纹。鬲通体饰三组兽面纹，足饰弦纹。清宫旧物（原藏颐和园）。

故宫博物院藏

The vessel is connected by a Zeng and a Li and a grate in the middle of the belly. The steamer has a flared mouth, two prick ears, and three hoof-shaped feet. The belly is decorated with close-grained setoff thunder pattern. The upper part is decorated with beast face patterns, and the lower part is covered with banana leaf-shaped Kui dragon designs (a one-legged monstrous animal in legend). The whole body of Li is designed with three groups of beast face patterns, and the feet are decorated with string patterns. The vessel belongs to the inner court of the imperial palace of the Qing Dynasty and was originally preserved in the Summer Palace. Preserved in The Palace Museum

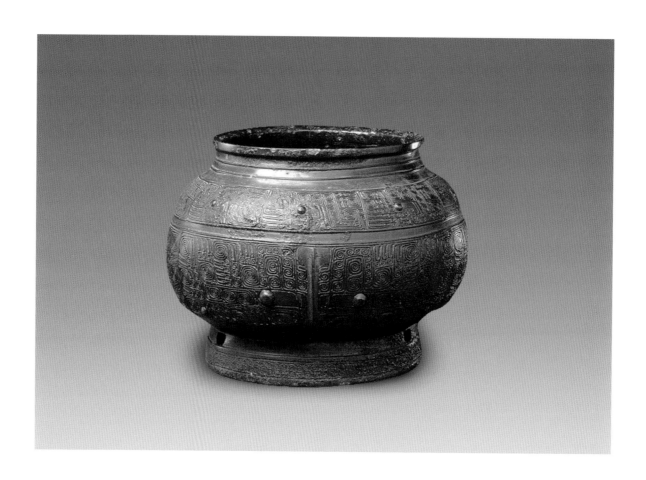

兽面纹瓿

商代晚期

青铜质

口径 16.1 厘米，宽 23.5 厘米，高 16.8 厘米，重 2.5 千克

Bu with Animal Mask Pattern

Late Shang Dynasty

Bronze

Mouth Diameter 16.1 cm/ Width 23.5 cm/ Height 16.8 cm/ Weight 2.5 kg

圆体，大腹，敛口，圈足。口沿下饰二道弦纹。腹部饰由各种形状的云雷纹组合成两种兽面纹。圈足饰云雷纹，有三个穿孔。清宫旧物（原藏颐和园）。

故宫博物院藏

This vessel has a round body, a big belly, a contracted mouth, and a ring foot. The vessel is decorated with two circles of string pattern under the mouth, and the belly, designed with two kinds of beast face patterns which are composed of cloud and thunder patterns in different shapes. The ring foot with three holes is covered with cloud and thunder pattern. The vessel belongs to the imperial palace of the Qing Dynasty and was originally preserved in the Summer Palace.

Preserved in The Palace Museum

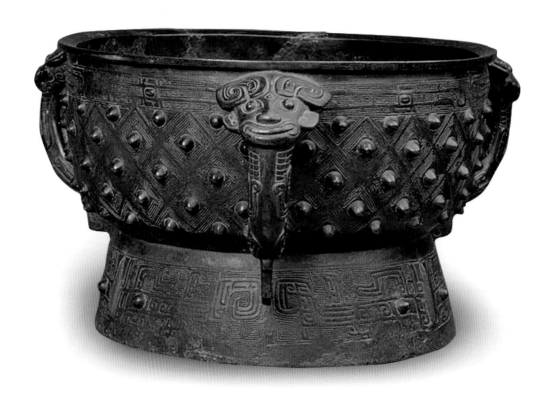

乳钉三耳簋

商代晚期

青铜质

口径 30.5 厘米，高 19.1 厘米，重 6.94 千克

Gui with Nipple Pattern and Three Looped Handles

Late Shang Dynasty

Bronze

Mouth Diameter 30.5 cm/ Height 19.1 cm/ Weight 6.94 kg

圆体，深腹，高圈足。口沿下线刻三圈目雷纹，腹部在菱形格纹地上饰乳丁纹。圈足微外撇，用柔和均匀的线条刻成三组兽面纹，以细密的雷纹为地。每组兽面纹的中心线准确地位于两耳之间。这种有规律的纹饰组合，具有浓厚的装饰色彩。耳呈兽形，雕刻精美，兽面部表情很生动。清宫旧物（原藏颐和园）。

故宫博物院藏

This vessel has a round body with a deep belly and a high ring foot. The upper part of the vessel is decorated with three circles of eye-like whorled patterns (eye-thunder pattern). On the belly, there is diamond-type lattice pattern as ground-tint over which there are nipple designs. The ring foot slightly extends outward and is decorated with three groups of beast face patterns using soft and well-distributed lines with fine-grained squared whorled patterns as the ground-tint. The central line of each group of the beast face patterns lies exactly between the two ears. This kind of organized combination of patterns and decorations achieves a strong sense of ornamentation. The exquisite ears are made into animal figures with vivid faces. This vessel belongs to the imperial palace of the Qing Dynasty and was originally kept in the Summer Palace.

Preserved in The Palace Museum

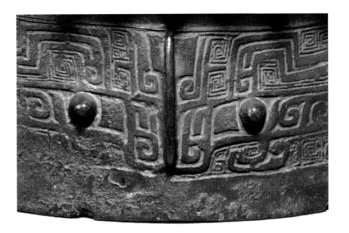

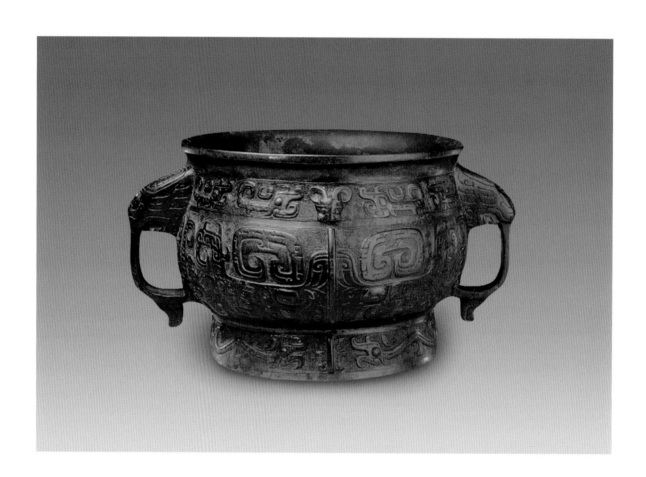

枚父辛簋

商代晚期

青铜质

宽 25.1 厘米，通高 18 厘米，重 5.36 千克

Gui with Characters "Mei Fu Xin"

Late Shang Dynasty

Bronze

Width 25.1 cm/ Height 18 cm/ Weight 5.36 kg

圆体，大腹，侈口，双兽耳，圈足。颈部前、
后各有一浮雕兽面。兽面两侧饰夔纹，腹饰
兽面纹，足饰夔纹，双耳内饰蝉纹。器外底
饰凸起的蟠龙纹，铭文"枚父辛"1行3字
在器内底。清宫旧藏。

故宫博物院藏

This vessel has a round body, a big belly, a
flared mouth, two ears with beast designs and
a ring foot. On the front and back sides of the
neck, there is a relief image of beast face on
each of them. Two sides of the beast face are
decorated with Kui dragon patterns, and the
belly is decorated with beast face patterns. The
foot is decorated with Kui dragon patterns, and
the inner areas of the two ears are decorated
with cicada designs. The outer bottom of the
vessel is decorated with convex patterns of
curled-up dragon. On the inner bottom of the
vessel, there is an inscription of 3 characters
in one line: "Mei Fu Xin". The vessel belongs
to the imperial palace of the Qing Dynasty and
was originally kept in the Summer Palace.
Preserved in The Palace Museum

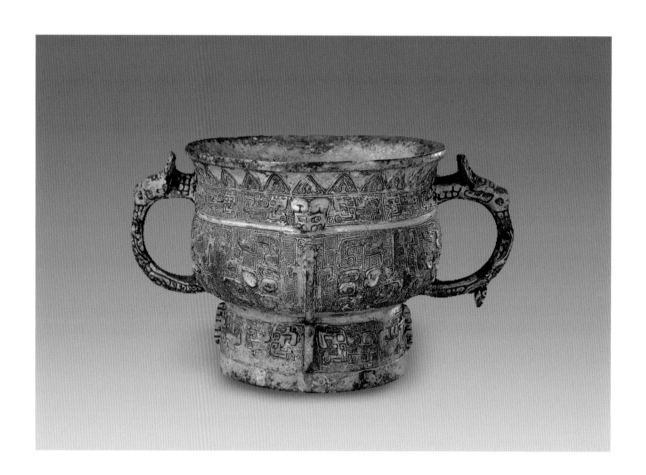

兽面纹簋

商代晚期

青铜质

宽 25.6 厘米，通高 14.1 厘米，重 1.62 千克

Gui with Animal Mask Pattern

Late Shang Dynasty

Bronze

Width 25.6 cm/ Height 14.1 cm/ Weight 1.62 kg

圆体，鼓腹，侈口，双兽耳，高圈足。腹前、后面上各有一凸棱，以凸棱为鼻饰兽面纹，口下饰齿形纹一圈，颈饰二浮雕兽面及夔纹，足饰夔纹及四凸棱。1946 年入藏。

故宫博物院藏

This is a food container. This vessel has a round body, a swelling belly, a flared mouth, two loop handles with beast designs, and a long ring foot. On the front and back sides of the belly, there each is a convex ridge, and the convex ridge is the nose with animal mask pattern. The lower part is decorated with a circle of tooth-like pattern. The neck is covered with two beast faces in relief and Kui dragon pattern, while the foot is decorated with Kui dragon pattern with four convex ridges. This container was collected in 1946.

Preserved in The Palace Museum

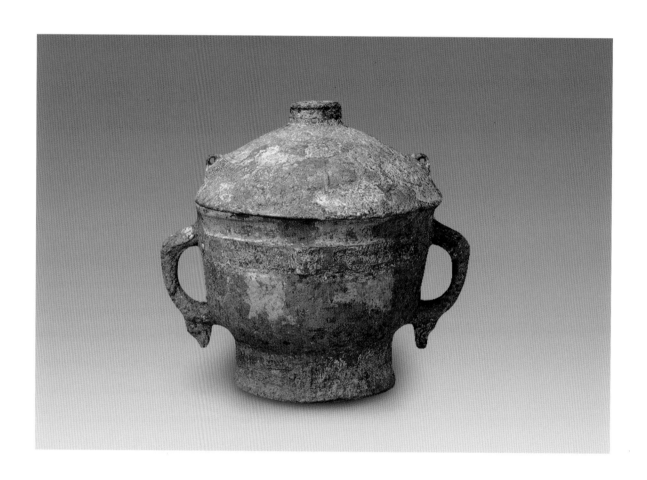

亚咠簋

商代晚期

青铜质

宽 26 厘米，通高 22.4 厘米，重 3.16 千克

Gui with Characters Including "咠"

Late Shang Dynasty

Bronze

Width 26 cm/ Height 22.4 cm/ Weight 3.16 kg

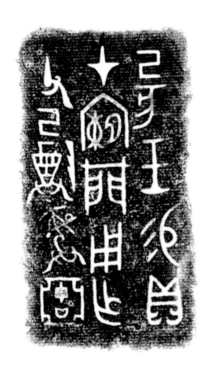

圆体，深腹，腹两侧各有一兽耳，圈足，有盖，盖顶正中有一圆握，上有二穿孔，握两侧各有一系。盖边、颈及足均饰夔纹组成的兽面纹，颈部前、后两面各饰一凸牺首。此簋盖、器对铭3行16字。传河南洛阳出土，章乃器先生捐献。

故宫博物院藏

This is a food container with a round body, a deep belly, a ring foot and a cover. On each of the two sides of the belly, there is a handle with designs of a beast. There is a cover, and in the center of the top of the cover, there is a round knob, and there are two pierced holes on the knob. On either side of the knob, there is a tie. The cover rim, the neck and the foot are decorated with beast face patterns made up of Kui dragon pattern. On the front and the back sides of the neck, there is a raised animal head. There is an inscription of 16 characters in 3 lines. It was said that this vessel was unearthed in Luoyang City, Henan Province and donated by Mr. Zhang Naiqi.

Preserved in The Palace Museum

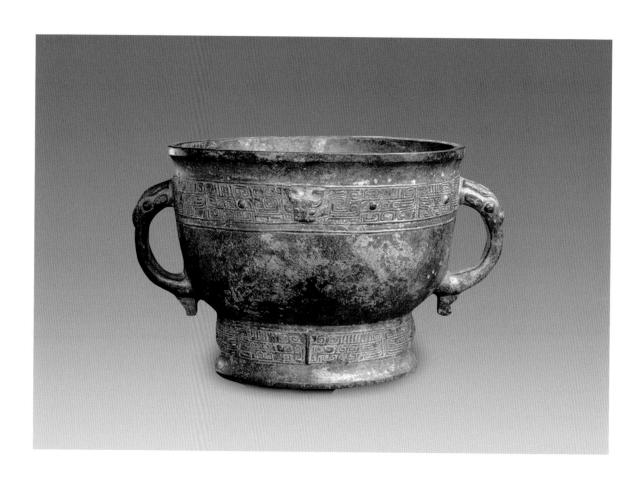

遽簋

商代晚期

青铜质

宽 25.5 厘米，通高 14.2 厘米，重 2 千克

Gui with Character "Li"

Late Shang Dynasty

Bronze

Width 25.5 cm/ Height 14.2 cm/ Weight 2 kg

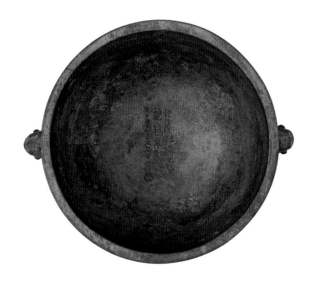

圆体，深腹，腹两侧各有一兽耳，圈足。颈部前、后两面各饰一凸兽首，周围饰夔纹及弦纹一周，足饰夔纹组成的兽面纹。器内底铭文 3 行 20 字。章乃器先生捐献。

故宫博物院藏

This is a food container with a round body, a deep belly and a ring foot. On the front and back sides of the neck, there is each a convex design of a head of a beast. Around the neck there is a circle of Kui dragon pattern and string pattern. There is a loop handle with a design of a beast on each side of the belly. The foot is designed with beast face pattern composed of Kui dragon pattern. On the bottom there is an inscription of 20 characters in 3 lines. This vessel was donated by Mr. Zhang Naiqi.
Preserved in The Palace Museum

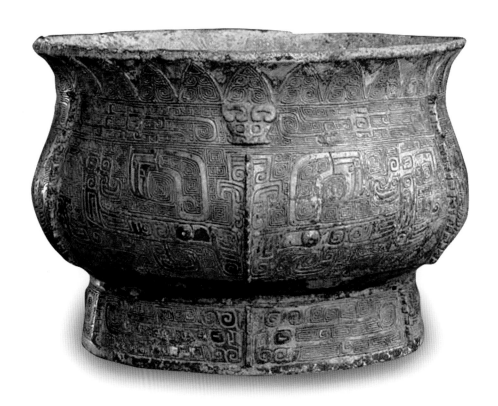

癸簋

商代晚期

青铜质

口径 12.8 厘米，高 12.7 厘米，重 1.78 千克

侈口，鼓腹，圈足。通体以雷纹为地。口沿下饰蕉叶纹、目雷纹。腹饰兽面纹，兽面双眼位置较低，前额宽大，正中雕一兽头。圈足饰以雷纹组成的兽面纹。器内有铭文"癸"2字。河南安阳出土，1960 年北京市文化局调拨。

故宫博物院藏

Gui with Characters Including "⊠"

Late Shang Dynasty

Bronze

Mouth Diameter 12.8 cm/ Height 12.7 cm/ Weight 1.78 kg

This is a food container. The vessel has a flared mouth, a swelling belly, and a ring foot. The whole body is decorated with squared whorled (thunder) pattern. There are banana leaf pattern and eye-like pattern along with thunder pattern. The belly is decorated with beast face pattern, and eyes of the beast with broad forehead are in the lower position which is carved with a beast head in the middle position. The ring foot is decorated with beast face pattern composed of thunder pattern. There is an inscription of 2 characters " ⊠ Kui" inside the vessel. This vessel was unearthed in Anyang County, Henan Province. It was allocated from Beijing Municipal Bureau of Culture in 1960.

Preserved in The Palace Museum

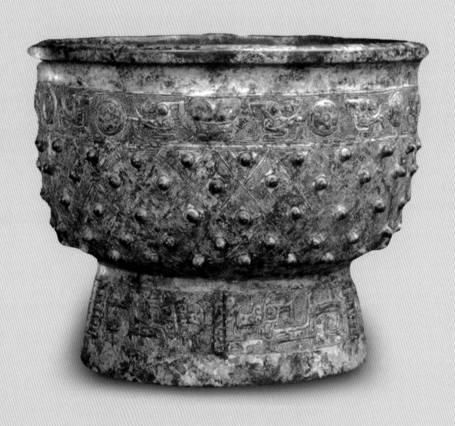

𰀨簋

商代晚期

青铜质

宽 24.9 厘米，通高 18.9 厘米，重 4.1 千克

圆体，深腹，方口沿，圈足，足上有六凸棱。颈饰
鸟纹间饰涡纹，腹饰菱形雷纹及乳丁，足饰鸟纹。
铭文一"𰀨"字在器内底。1946 年入藏。

故宫博物院藏

Gui with Character "𰀨"

Late Shang Dynasty

Bronze

Width 24.9 cm/ Height 18.9 cm/ Weight 4.1 kg

This is a food container with a round body, a deep belly,
a square-edged mouth, and a ring foot. There are six
convex ridges on the foot. The neck is decorated with
sectioned pattern of bird and vortex pattern. The belly
is decorated with diamond-shaped thunder pattern and
nipple design. The foot is decorated with bird pattern.
On the inner part of the bottom, there is an inscription
of one character " 𰀨 ". This vessel was collected in
1946.

Preserved in The Palace Museum

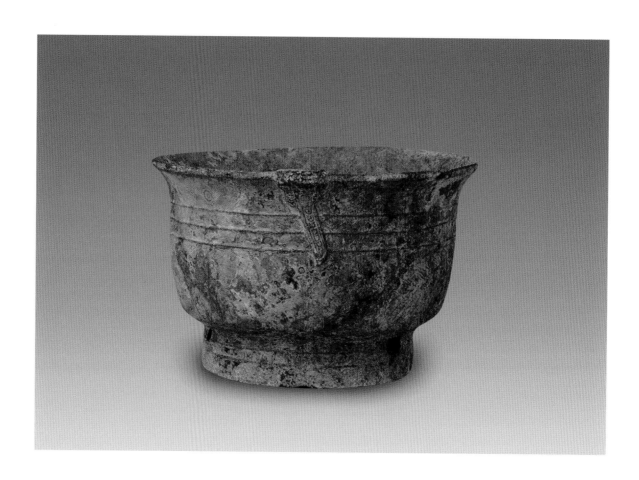

专簋

商代晚期

青铜质

宽 20.6 厘米，通高 12.8 厘米，重 1.8 千克

Gui with Character "Zhuan"

Late Shang Dynasty

Bronze

Width 20.6 cm/ Height 12.8 cm/ Weight 1.8 kg

圆体，深腹，侈口，圈足。颈饰弦纹三圈，足饰弦纹二圈，口内外各有一条形补痕，上饰夔纹。铭文一"专"字在器内。口上的补痕为原补，当时为了美观，把青铜补片做成夔形。1956 年国家文物局调拨。

故宫博物院藏

This is a food container with a round body, a deep belly, a flared mouth and a ring foot. The neck is decorated with three circles of string patterns and the foot with two circles of string patterns. There is a mending mark both inside and outside the mouth, each of which is decorated with Kui dragon pattern. On the inside of the vessel, there is an inscription of one character "Zhuan". The mending marks inside and outside the mouth are the original marks. It is presumed that the bronze pieces were shaped in Kui dragon form for aesthetic purpose. This vessel was allocated from State Administration of Cultural Heritage in 1956. Preserved in The Palace Museum

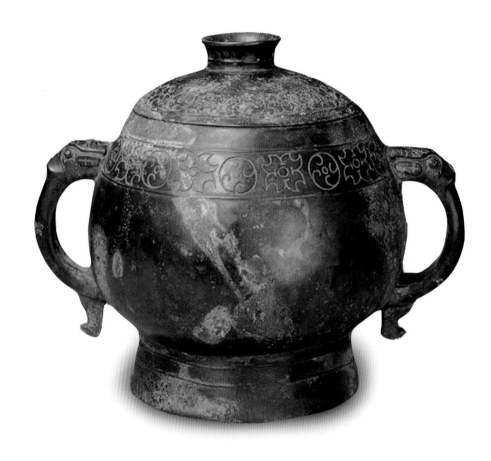

亚醜父丁簋

商代晚期

青铜质

宽 30 厘米，通高 23.3 厘米，重 4.44 千克

体圆似球形，深腹，敛口，圈足。腹两侧各有一兽耳，盖上有一圆握，握上有二方穿孔。盖、肩及器口下均饰涡纹，间饰四瓣花纹，足饰弦纹二道，器外底有一凸起四瓣花纹。器内底有铭文 1 行 4 字。1961 年国家文物局调拨。

故宫博物院藏

Gui with Four Characters Including "醜"

Late Shang Dynasty

Bronze

Width 30 cm/ Height 23.3 cm/ Weight 4.44 kg

This is a food container. This round-bodied pot which is like a ball has a deep belly, a convergent mouth and a ring foot. There is a handle on both sides of the belly with beast design. There is a knob on the cover with two square holes. The lower part of the cover, the shoulder and the mouth are decorated with whorled patterns and in between with a flower pattern composed of four petals. The foot is decorated with two circles of string patterns. There is a convex quatrefoil-like pattern on the outer bottom of the vessel. On the inner bottom, there is an inscription of 4 characters in one line. This vessel was allocated from State Administration of Cultural Heritage in 1961.

Preserved in The Palace Museum

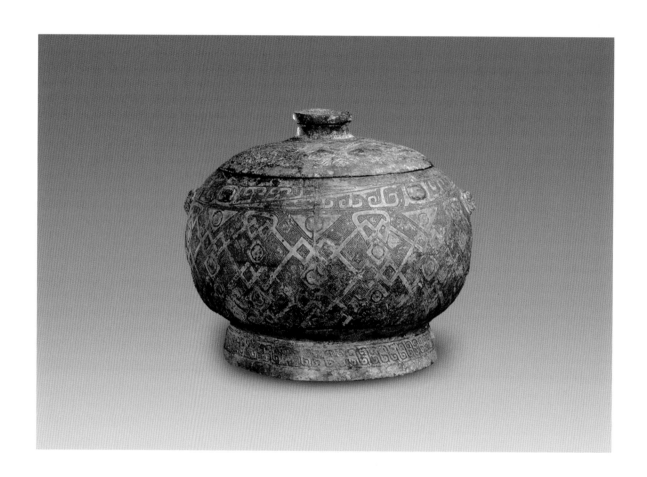

▨簋

商代晚期

青铜质

宽 21.2 厘米，通高 17.4 厘米，重 2.7 千克

Gui with Character "▨"

Late Shang Dynasty

Bronze

Width 21.2 cm/ Height 17.4 cm/ Weight 2.7 kg

球形体，平口，圈足。肩部有双贯耳，盖有子口，盖顶上有一圆握，握有二穿孔。盖饰勾连雷纹，颈饰斜角目雷纹，腹饰斜方格勾连目雷纹，足饰雷纹。器内底及盖内均有一"▨"字。传河南安阳出土，1946 年入藏。

故宫博物院藏

This vessel has a ball-shaped body, a flat mouth and a ring foot. There are two pierced ears on the shoulder, and there is a matching mouth on the cover. There is a round knob with two pierced holes on the top of the cover. The cover is decorated with intertwined thunder pattern and the neck with oblique eye-like pattern surrounded by thunder pattern. The belly is decorated with oblique diamond-shaped intertwined eye-like pattern surrounded by thunder pattern. The foot is decorated with thunder pattern. There is a character "▨" both on the inside of the bottom and the inner side of the cover. It is said that this vessel was unearthed in Anyang City, Henan Province and was collected in 1946.

Preserved in The Palace Museum

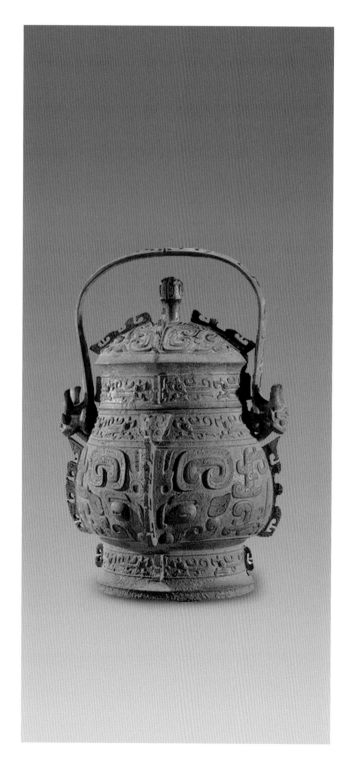

"烎作父丁"饕餮纹铜卣

商代晚期

青铜质

通高 40 厘米

**Bronze You with Tao Tie Pattern
and Characters Including " 烎 "**

Late Shang Dynasty

Bronze

Height 40 cm

子母口，圆腹，圈足。器侧面附有提梁。有盖，盖顶有一菌形钮。盖和器身四面有扉棱，无地纹，盖的顶面及腹部饰饕餮纹，盖的下部、肩和圈足饰夔纹，提梁两端饰兽头。盖和器身均有铭文"𠦪(作父丁宝尊彝"7字。

河北博物院藏

The vessel has a snap lid mouth, a round belly, a ring foot, a loop handle on its flanks, and a cover with a mushroom-like knob. The four sides of the cover and the vessel are cast with flanges, but without ground-tint. The top area of the cover and the belly are decorated with Tao Tie (a mythical ferocious animal) pattern. The lower part of the cover, the shoulder and the ring foot of the vessel are decorated with Kui dragon design. The two ends of the loop handle are adorned with animal heads. There is an inscription on both the cover and the body of the vessel: an inscription of 7 characters including " 𠦪(Zuo Fu Ding Bao Zun Yi".
Preserved in Hebei Museum

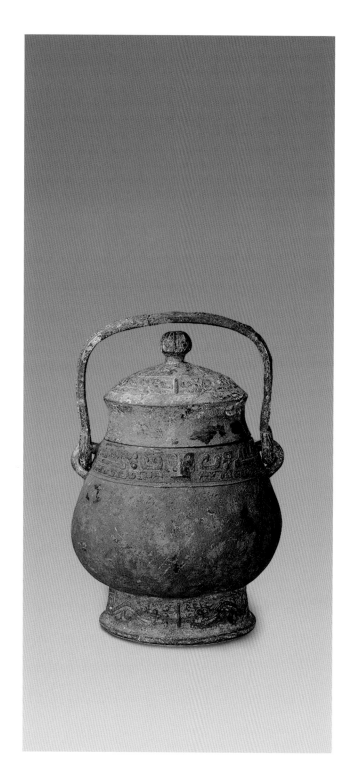

二祀邲其卣

商代晚期

青铜质

宽 36.9 厘米，通高 38.4 厘米，重 8.86 千克

You with Characters Including "邲"

Late Shang Dynasty

Bronze

Width 36.9 cm/ Height 38.4 cm/ Weight 8.86 kg

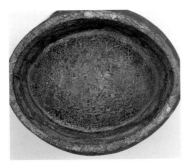

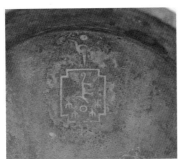

椭圆体，短颈，两侧有环，套铸提梁，鼓腹，圈足外侈。有盖，上饰菌形握。颈前、后各饰一兽首。盖沿、颈、足均饰夔纹。盖与器内均有铭文"亚貘父丁"。器外底铸 7 行 39 字。河南安阳出土，1946 年入藏。

故宫博物院藏

The vessel is oval in shape with a short neck, a ring on both sides interlinked with the loop handle, a swelling belly, an ring foot that tilts outwardly, and a cover with a mushroom-like knob. A beast head is adorned on both the front and the back of the neck. Kui dragon design is decorated on the cover edge, the neck, and the ring foot. The inscription on the cover and the body is "Ya Mo Fu Ding". The outer bottom is inscribed with 39 characters in 7 lines. The vessel was excavated from Anyang City, Henan Province, and was collected in 1946.

Preserved in The Palace Museum

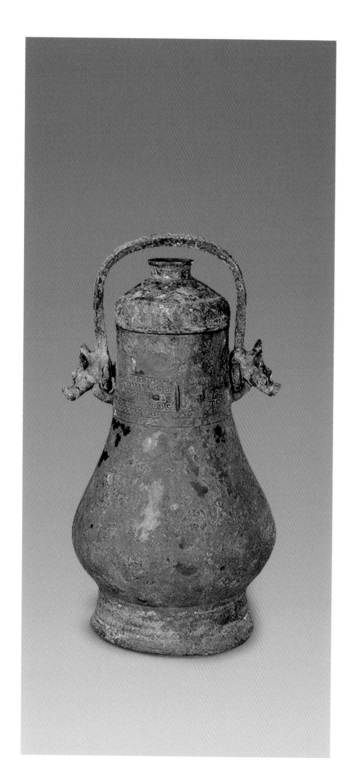

四祀弋其卣

商代晚期

青铜质

宽 19.3 厘米，通高 34.5 厘米，重 4.2 千克

You with Characters Including "弋其"

Late Shang Dynasty

Bronze

Width 19.3 cm/ Height 34.5 cm/ Weight 4.2 kg

圆体，长颈，两侧有环，套铸双兽头梁，腹深且下垂，圈足外侈。盖上有圆形握。盖、梁、足均饰雷纹，颈饰兽面纹。盖与器内有"亚貘父丁"四字。器外底铸铭文 8 行 42 字。河南安阳出土，1956 年收购。

故宫博物院藏

The vessel has a round body, a long neck, a ring on both sides interlinked with loop handle with double beast heads, a deep and droopy belly, a ring foot that tilts outwardly, and a lid with a round knob. The thunder pattern is designed on the cover, the loop handle and the ring foot. The neck is decorated with animal mask pattern. There is an inscription of 4 characters "Ya Mo Fu Ding" on the cover and inner body of the vessel. The outer bottom of the vessel is inscribed with 42 characters in 8 lines. The vessel was excavated from Anyang City, Henan Province, and acquired in 1946.
Preserved in The Palace Museum

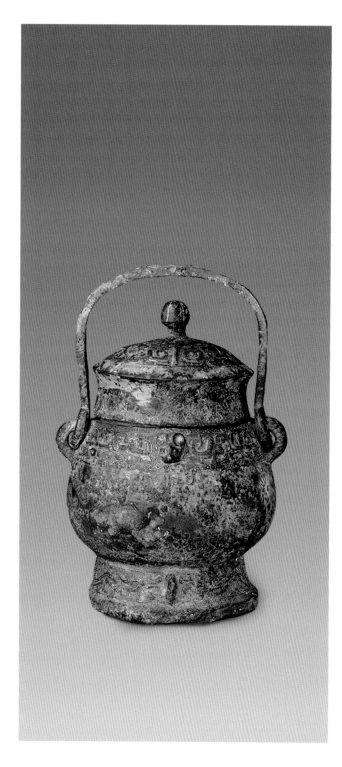

六祀邲其卣

商代晚期

青铜质

宽 15.7 厘米，通高 23.7 厘米，重 1.98 千克

You with Characters Including "邲"

Late Shang Dynasty

Bronze

Width 15.7 cm/ Height 23.7 cm/ Weight 1.98 kg

椭圆体，短颈，鼓腹，圈足外撇，颈两侧环耳内套铸提梁。有盖，盖顶圆拱，上有一菌状握。盖、梁、腹、足均饰夔纹，颈饰 2 个对称的牺首。盖与器对铭，各有铭文 5 行 29 字。河南安阳出土，1957 年收购。

故宫博物院藏

The oval vessel has a short neck, a swelling belly, a ring foot that tilts outwardly, a ring ear on both sides of the neck interlinked with the loop handle, and a dome-shaped cover with a mushroom-like knob. Kui design is decorated on the cover, the loop handle, the belly and the ring foot. The neck is adorned with two symmetric animal heads. The inscription on the cover corresponds with that of the body of the vessel, an inscription of 29 characters in 5 lines. The vessel was excavated from Anyang City, Henan Province, and acquired in 1957.

Preserved in The Palace Museum

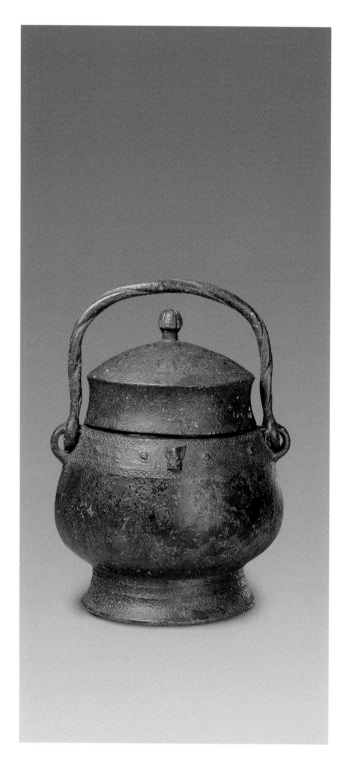

子卣

商代晚期

青铜质

宽 22.5 厘米，通高 28 厘米，重 3.84 千克

You with Character "Zi"

Late Shang Dynasty

Bronze

Width 22.5 cm/ Height 28 cm/ Weight 3.84 kg

椭圆形体，提梁呈纽索状。盖顶和器颈均饰兽面纹。颈部有牺首相隔。盖与器对铭，各有铭文 3 行 15 字。清宫旧物（原藏颐和园）。

故宫博物院藏

The vessel is oval in shape with a rope-like loop handle. The top of the cover and the neck of the vessel are adorned with animal mask designs. The neck is divided into two sections with an animal head. There is an inscription of 15 characters in 3 lines on both the cover and the body of the vessel, and they correspond with each other. It is an antique from the imperial palace of the Qing Dynasty (originally kept in the Summer Palace).

Preserved in The Palace Museum

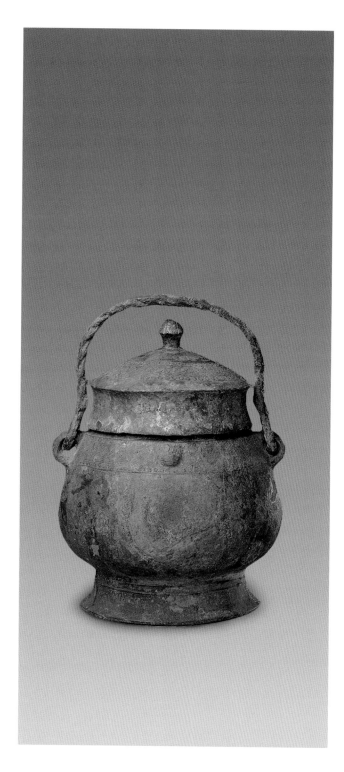

孤竹卣

商代晚期

青铜质

宽 24.3 厘米，通高 32 厘米，重 5 千克

You with Characters "Gu Zhu"

Late Shang Dynasty

Bronze

Width 24.3 cm/ Height 32 cm/ Weight 5 kg

鼓腹，圈足。盖上有圆钉帽状钮，肩有双耳，

中有提梁。盖顶饰夔纹，口下饰夔纹和一对

兽首。盖内和器底均有铭 7 字。1954 年收购。

　　　　　　　　　　　　故宫博物院藏

The vessel has a swelling belly and a ring foot.
The cover has a round pin-like knob in the
shape of a cap, a pair of ears on the shoulder, a
loop handle in the middle of the vessel, There
is Kui dragon pattern on the top of the cover.
The rim below the mouth is decorated with
Kui dragon pattern and a pair of beast heads.
The inner side of the cover and the bottom of
the vessel are inscribed with 7 characters. The
vessel was acquired in 1954.

Preserved in The Palace Museum

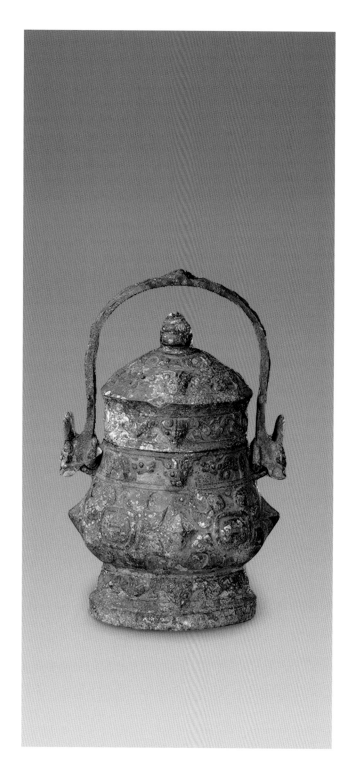

牛纹卣

商代晚期

青铜质

宽 23 厘米，高 29.5 厘米，重 3.62 千克

You with Ox Pattern

Late Shang Dynasty

Bronze

Width 23 cm/ Height 29.5 cm/ Weight 3.62 kg

椭圆形体，有盖，圈足，活络提梁。通体纹饰，盖钮呈盘蛇状，提梁的两端做成兽头形。纹饰从提梁至圈足共有六层，其中提梁、口沿下、圈足均饰兽头双身纹，兽头位于正中，双身向左右伸展。盖、颈部饰牛纹。两牛之间饰一兽头，与兽头双身纹中的兽头同位于卣身的纵向中心线上。1956 年国家文物局调拨。

故宫博物院藏

The oval vessel has a cover, a ring foot, and a movable loop handle. The whole body is adorned with decorative patterns. The knob on the cover is designed as a coiled snake and the two ends of the loop handle are made into a shape of an animal head. There are six layers of decorative patterns from the loop handle to the ring foot, among which patterns of animal heads with double bodies are decorated on the loop handle, the rim area below the mouth and the ring foot (with the animal head in the center and the double bodies extend to the right and left), while the ox pattern is decorated on the cover and the neck. Between two oxen is an animal head, which is on the longitudinal center line of the body, same with that of the animal head in the compound animal pattern. This vessel was allocated from State Administration of Cultural Heritage in 1956.

Preserved in The Palace Museum

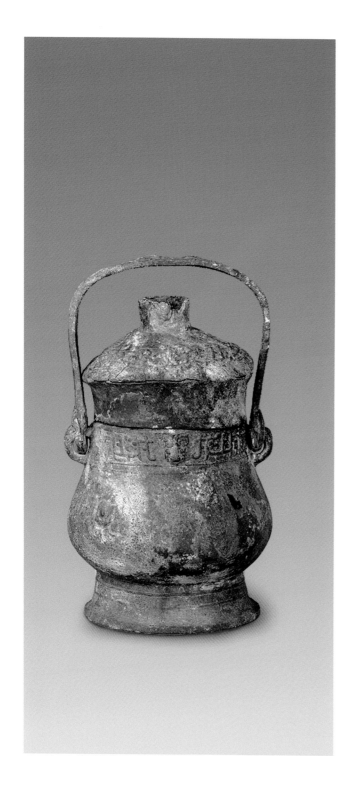

处山卣

商代晚期

青铜质

宽 16.2 厘米，通高 26.2 厘米，重 3.34 千克

You with Characters Including "处"

Late Shang Dynasty

Bronze

Width 16.2 cm/ Height 26.2 cm/ Weight 3.34 kg

椭圆形体，鼓腹，圈足。隆盖，盖冠呈圈状。肩有双耳，中有提梁。盖顶和器颈均饰回首夔纹，颈部中隔浮雕兽首，圈足饰两道弦纹。盖、器对铭，各铸 25 字。1954 年国家文物局调拨。

故宫博物院藏

The vessel is oval in shape with a swelling belly, a ring foot, a raised cover with its crest area in the shape of circles. There are two ears on the shoulder, and the hoop handle is in the middle of the vessel. The top of the cover and the neck are adorned with pattern of Kui dragon looking back. The middle of the neck is divided into two sections by a decoration of an animal head in relief. Two streaks of string pattern are decorated on the ring foot. The inscription on the cover is the same as that on the vessel, with 25 characters for both inscriptions. This vessel was allocated from State Administration of Cultural Heritage in 1954.

Preserved in The Palace Museum

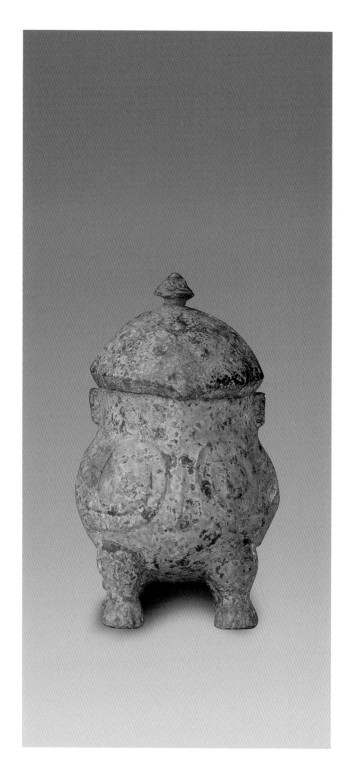

葡贝鸮卣

商代晚期

青铜质

宽 14.2 厘米，通高 17.1 厘米，重 1.18 千克

You with Characters Including "葡"

Late Shang Dynasty

Bronze

Width 14.2 cm/ Height 17.1 cm/ Weight 1.18 kg

卣呈两鸮相背形。钮帽菌形，上饰云纹。腹饰鸮翼纹，器两侧口下设提梁，而增饰浮雕兽首，四矮兽足。盖内和器底均有铭文 2 字："茜贝"。1946 年入藏。

故宫博物院藏

The vessel is in the shape of two back-to-back owls, and its cover knob is mushroom-like with decorative cloud pattern and the belly is adorned with owl-feather pattern. There is no loop handle for this vessel, but an animal head in relief is decorated in the area under the rim of the mouth on both sides of the belly. The vessel has four short feet in the shape of an animal. There is an inscription of 2 characters both on the inner side of the cover and the bottom of the vessel. This vessel was collected in 1946.

Preserved in The Palace Museum

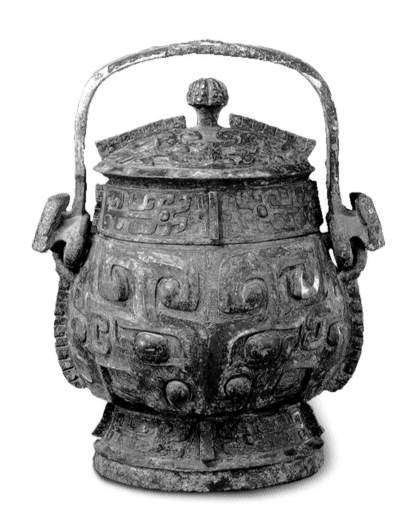

𫛭父乙卣

商代晚期

青铜质

宽 27.7 厘米，通高 31.4 厘米，重 6.2 千克

器的四面皆出棱脊，给人以凝重之感。提梁两端饰兽头。全器以纤细的云雷纹为地，盖顶与器腹为大兽面，双目特大；盖沿与圈足饰夔纹。盖、器对铭，各有铭文 4 字。1946 年入藏。

故宫博物院藏

You with Characters Including "𫛭"

Late Shang Dynasty

Bronze

Width 27.7 cm/ Height 31.4 cm/ Weight 6.2 kg

This vessel has ridges on its four sides, making it look dignified. Both ends of the loop handle are decorated with the design of an animal head. There are fine cloud and thunder patterns on the surface of the whole vessel as the ground-tint. The top of the cover and the belly are decorated with large animal masks with especially big eyes. The cover edge and the ring foot are decorated with Kui dragon pattern. The cover and the body of the vessel have the same inscription of 4 characters respectively. It was collected in 1946.

Preserved in The Palace Museum

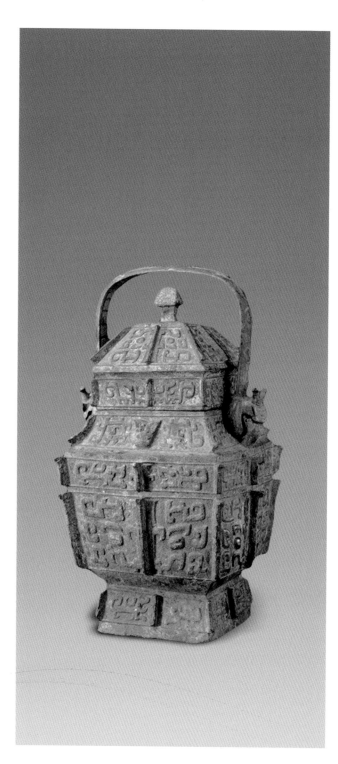

屮册父戊方卣

商代晚期

青铜质

宽 21.5 厘米，通高 38 厘米，重 5.78 千克

Square You with Characters Including "屮册"

Late Shang Dynasty

Bronze

Width 21.5 cm/ Height 38 cm/ Weight 5.78 kg

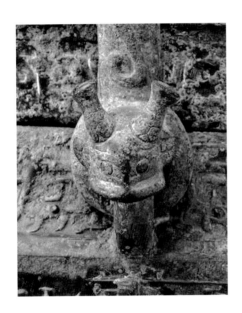

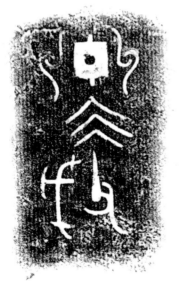

方形，平底，直颈。盖顶设屋宇形钮。盖饰兽面纹，盖口的夔龙呈回首垂冠形。肩部的纹饰为团身夔纹，中隔牺首，肩两侧置兽首提梁。腹部纹饰分为两部分，上部饰两两相对的夔纹，下部饰分解状的兽面纹。盖与器内铸有7字对铭。1946年入藏。

故宫博物院藏

This wine vessel has a rectangular shape with a flat bottom and a straight neck. The knob on the top of the cover is shaped like a building with a peak roof. There is decoration of animal mask pattern on the cover. The decoration of Kui dragon on the cover mouth is designed to turn its head back with dropping crest. The pattern on the shoulder is a coiled Kui dragon. Between the shoulders there is a beast head design. The vessel has a loop handle with an animal head on each of its ends. The upper part of the belly is decorated with patterns of two Kui dragons that look face to face, and the lower part with decomposed beast face mask. The same inscription of 7 characters is inscribed on the cover and the inner side of the vessel. This vessel was collected in 1946.

Preserved in The Palace Museum

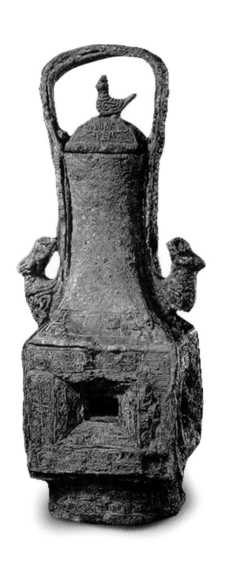

十字洞腹方卣

商代晚期

青铜质

口径 6.6 厘米，宽 15 厘米，高 34.5 厘米，

重 3.54 千克

Square You with a Crisscross Square Hole

Late Shang Dynasty

Bronze

Mouth Diameter 6.6 cm/ Width 15 cm/ Height

34.5 cm/ Weight 3.54 kg

长颈，方腹，圈足。盖钮呈一立鸟状。盖通体饰兽面纹，一侧饰有蝉纹，蝉尾跷起处有一圆孔，与提梁上的孔之间原有链相连。肩两侧各饰一伏鸟，两鸟尾上卷相连形成提梁。肩角处各饰一组兽面纹，足饰目雷纹。腹部在细密的雷纹地上饰兽面纹及目纹。方腹正中有十字形方孔，四面相通。北京市文化局调拨。

故宫博物院藏

This vessel is characterized by a long neck, a square belly, and a ring foot. The knob of the cover is shaped like a standing bird. There are animal mask patterns on the whole cover. One side of the cover is decorated with cicada patterns, and on the area where the tail of the cicada rises there is a round hole originally connected with the hole on the hoop handle with a chain. The both sides of the shoulder are decorated with a prostrate bird with its tail curling up to form the hoop handle. There is a group of animal mask patterns on each side of the shoulder, and eye-like pattern with square whorled pattern decorated with the ring foot. The fine animal mask pattern and eye-like pattern are decorated on the found-tint of thunder pattern on the belly. There is a square hole in the shape of a cross on each side of the belly that can communicate from all sides. This vessel was allocated from Beijing Municipal Bureau of Culture.

Preserved in The Palace Museum

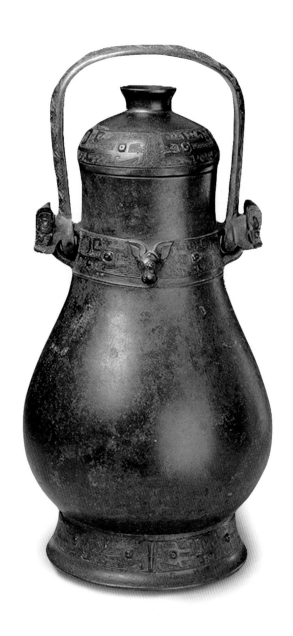

鸢祖辛卣

商代晚期

青铜质

宽 18.4 厘米，通高 36.4 厘米，重 4.04 千克

细颈，腹下部鼓出，圈足。盖有捉手。提梁两端呈兽首形。

盖面、器颈和圈足均饰兽面纹，器颈在兽面中间加饰小兽首。

盖、器对铭，各铸铭文 3 字。清宫旧物（原藏颐和园）。

故宫博物院藏

You with Characters "Yuan Zu Xin"

Late Shang Dynasty

Bronze

Width 18.4 cm/ Height 36.4 cm/ Weight 4.04 kg

The vessel has a narrow neck, a belly with its lower part raising outward, and a ring foot. There is a knob on the cover. Both ends of the hoop handle are decorated like an animal head. Animal mask patterns are decorated on the surface of the cover, the neck and the ring foot. Located among the animal mask patterns, designs of little animal heads are added to the neck. There is the same inscription of 3 characters on the cover and the body of the vessel. This item is an antique of the imperial palace of the Qing Dynasty (originally collected in the Summer Palace).

Preserved in The Palace Museum

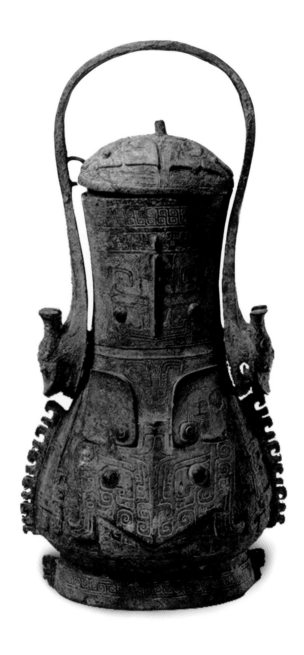

兽面纹卣

商代晚期

青铜质

宽 15.9 厘米，通高 25.3 厘米，重 2.32 千克

器身两面各饰凸雕的大兽面纹。宽额竖耳，形象比较特殊。颈上有提梁，两端呈龙头形。1956 年国家文物局调拨。

故宫博物院藏

You with Animal Mask Pattern

Late Shang Dynasty

Bronze

Width 15.9 cm/ Height 25.3 cm/ Weight 2.32 kg

Two sides of the body of the vessel are decorated with large animal mask patterns in relief. The beast are designed in a special way with broad forehead and prick ears. There is a hoop handle on the neck with both ends decorated with a dragon head. This vessel was allocated from State Administration of Cultural Heritage in 1956.

Preserved in The Palace Museum

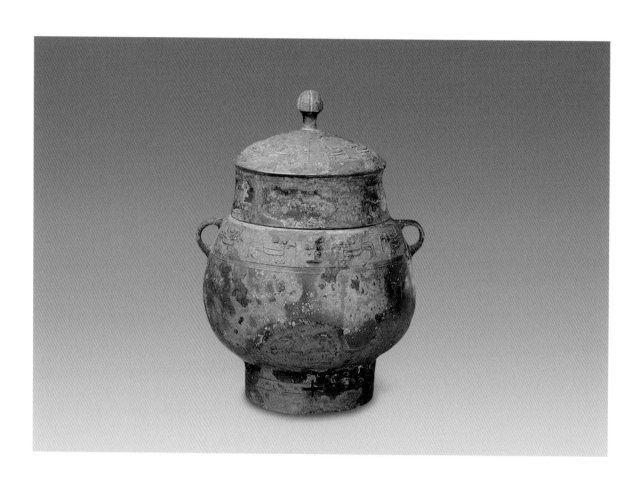

亚醶卣

商代晚期

青铜质

宽 22.3 厘米，通高 30 厘米，重 3.9 千克

You with Characters Including "醶"

Late Shang Dynasty

Bronze

Width 22.3 cm/ Height 30 cm/ Weight 3.9 kg

器体扁圆而丰满，肩、腹自然过渡，双环耳，圈足。有盖，上有一菌形握。盖沿饰鸟纹，腹饰鸟纹和对称的两个牺首，足饰弦纹，有十字孔。盖、器对铭。冀朝鼎先生捐献。

故宫博物院藏

This vessel has a flattened circular and plump body, two ring-shaped ears and a ring foot. The shoulder and the belly are naturally integrated. There is a knob on the cover shaped like a mushroom. There are bird patterns on the edge of the cover. There are bird patterns and designs of two symmetrical animal heads on the belly, and string pattern and cruciform holes on the ring foot. The same inscription is inscribed on the cover and the body of the vessel. It was donated by Mr. Ji Chaoding.

Preserved in The Palace Museum

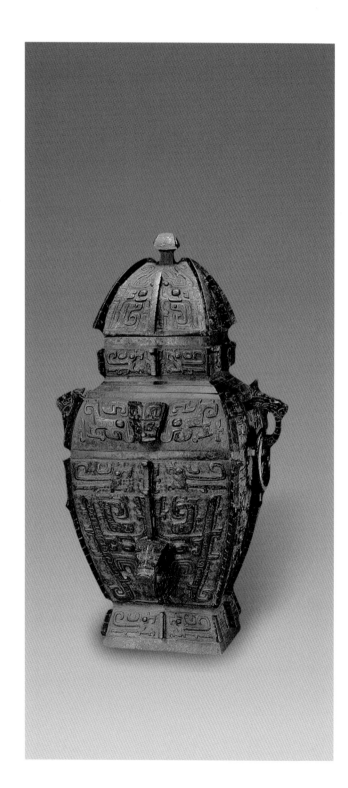

亚𠦪方罍

商代晚期

青铜质

宽 37.6 厘米，通高 60.8 厘米，重 20.8 千克

Lei with Characters Including "𠦪"

Late Shang Dynasty

Bronze

Width 37.6 cm/ Height 60.8 cm/ Weight 20.8 kg

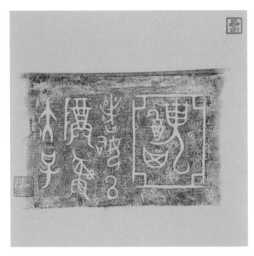

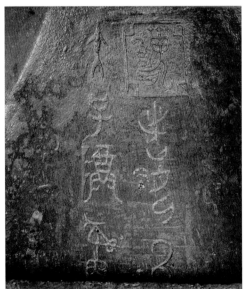

方体，鼓腹，方口，方圈足，肩两侧各有一兽首衔环，正背两面各有一浮雕兽首，腹部下有一兽首鋬，盖呈屋顶状，顶上一钮。盖、颈、腹足均饰八凸棱，钮、盖、腹均饰兽面纹，颈、肩、足饰夔纹。盖、器9字对铭，盖2行，器4行。清宫旧藏。

故宫博物院藏

This vessel has a square body, drum abdomen straight mouth and square ring foot. Flanks of the shoulder are decorated with designs of animal heads with ring in their mouth. The front and back of the shoulder are decorated with an animal head in relief. There is a handle shaped like an animal head Under the belly. The cover is like a roof top, with a knob on it. Eight decorative vertical ridges arc, in relief, cast on the cover, the neck, the shoulder, the belly and the foot. There are animal mask patterns on the cover, the should, and the belly, and there are Kui dragon patterns on the neck and foot. There is an inscription of 9 characters is 2 lines on the cover in 4 lines on the body. It used to be an antique of the imperial palace of the Qing Dynasty.

Preserved in The Palace Museum

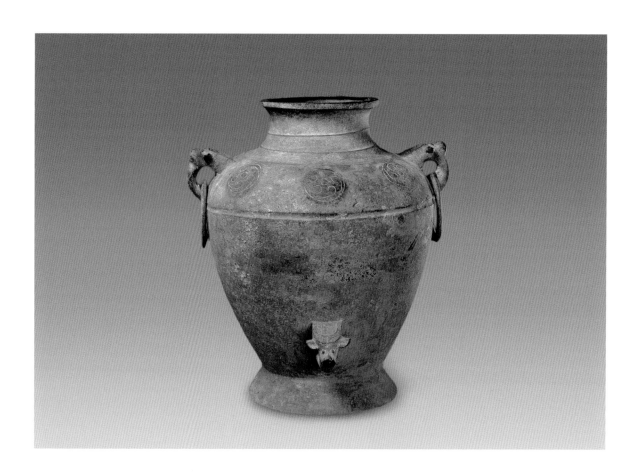

乃孙祖甲罍

商代晚期

青铜质

口径 18 厘米，宽 39 厘米，高 41.8 厘米，重 11.34 千克

Lei with Characters "Nai Sun Zu Jia"

Late Shang Dynasty

Bronze

Mouth Diameter 18 cm/ Width 39 cm/ Height 41.8 cm/ Weight 11.34 kg

圆体，直颈，侈口，平沿，广肩，圈足。颈部饰两道弦纹，肩部饰双兽首衔环，衔环间饰 6 个凸起的圆涡纹，腹下部有兽首鼻，口内壁有铭文 3 行 17 字。1956 年 12 月收购。

故宫博物院藏

This vessel has a round body, a straight neck, a wide flared mouth with flat edges, broad shoulders and a ring foot. The shoulder is decorated with designs of double animal heads holding rings in their mouths. There are two streaks of string patterns on the neck, and six raised patterns on the shoulder. On the lower part of the belly, there are decorations of noses of the animal heads. The inner wall of the mouth is inscribed with 17 characters in 3 lines. It was acquired in December 1956.

Preserved in The Palace Museum

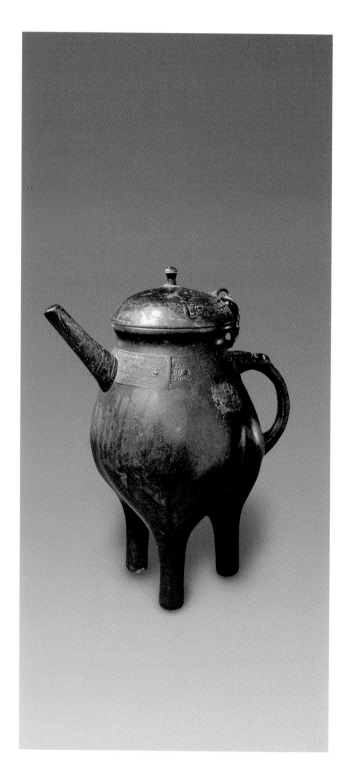

亚鸟宁盉

商代晚期

青铜质

宽 12.5 厘米，通高 31 厘米，重 3.86 千克

He with Characters "Ya Niao Ning"

Late Shang Dynasty

Bronze

Width 12.5 cm/ Height 31 cm/ Weight 3.86 kg

圆体，深腹，束颈，侈口。腹上有兽首鋬，颈部有一管状流，腹下三柱足，盖顶有一菌形钮，盖与器有链连接。盖、颈均饰兽面纹一周。有铭文 2 行 6 字。1956 年入藏。

故宫博物院藏

The vessel body is round in shape with a deep belly, a convergent neck, and a flare mouth. On the belly, there is a handle in the shape of the head of a sacred animal. On the neck, there is a tubular spout. Below the belly, there are three legs. There is a mushroom-shaped knob on the top of the cover, and the cover is joined to the vessel body with a chain. There is a circle of beast face pattern both on the cover and on the neck. There is an inscription of 6 characters in 2 lines on the vessel. The vessel was collected in 1956.

Preserved in The Palace Museum

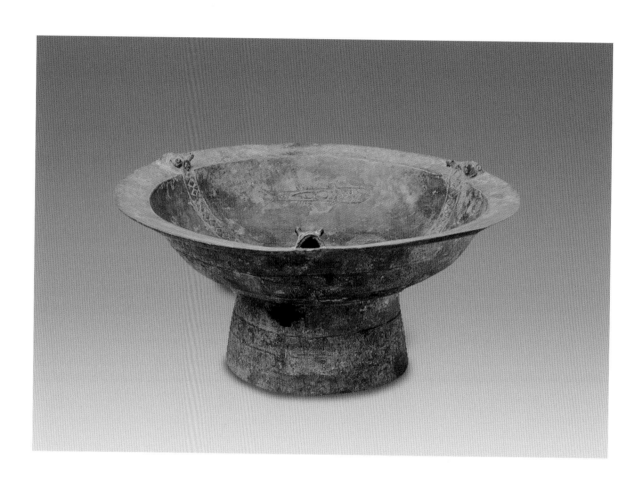

龟鱼龙纹盘

商代晚期

青铜质

口径 44 厘米，足径 19.7 厘米，高 19.2 厘米，重 4.78 千克

Plate with Designs of Turtle, Fish and Dragon

Late Shang Dynasty

Bronze

Calibre 44 cm/ Leg Diameter 19.7 cm/ Height 19.2 cm/ Weight 4.78 kg

圆体，浅腹，高圈足。盘的中心刻一龟纹，由盘底沿内壁向口沿的方向刻龙纹三条，龙身饰菱形纹，龙头浮在口沿上。在三条龙纹之间刻有三尾游鱼。三种纹饰均采用单线刻。盘外腹饰斜角回纹一圈，足饰回纹。圈足上有三个十字形穿孔。1946 年入藏。

故宫博物院藏

The round plate has a shallow belly and a high ring foot. The center of the plate is decorated with turtle design. From the bottom of the plate extending towards its rim, there are three lines of dragon design carved on it. These dragons are decorated with lozenge patterns, the dragon head is designed to float on the rim. Three fish are carved on the interval space of the three dragon designs. The three types of pattern are made in single lines. The exterior belly is decorated with a circle of rectangural spiral pattern with oblique angles. The foot is also decorated with fret pattern. On the ring foot, there are three crisscross holes. It was collected in 1946.

Preserved in The Palace Museum

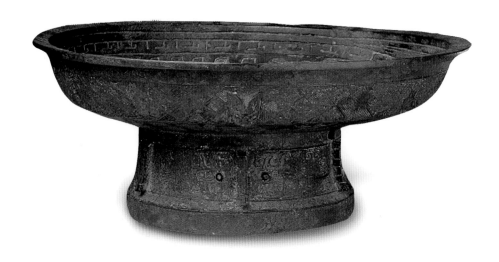

亚炅盘

商代晚期

青铜质

宽 35.3 厘米，通高 12.8 厘米，重 4.24 千克

Plate with Characters "Ya Yi"

Late Shang Dynasty

Bronze

Width 35.3 cm/ Height 12.8 cm/ Weight 4.24 kg

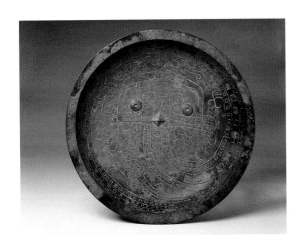

圆形，折沿，高圈足。盘内饰龙纹，龙首居中，身尾盘绕其外。外腹部饰雷纹带，并饰三只浮雕兽头。圈足上部有三个等距离的较大圆形孔，圈足下部在云雷纹地上饰了三组兽面纹，中间隔以扉棱。盘内底龙首处有铭文"亚㐭"二字。1958年收购。

故宫博物院藏

The round plate has folded edges and a high ring foot. The plate is decorated with dragon design, with the dragon head in the center and the tail coiling outside. The exterior of the belly is decorated with belts of cloud and thunder pattern and three relief sculptures in the shape of a beast head. On the ring foot, there are three big round holes, which are equidistant from each other. On the lower part of the foot, there are three groups of beast face pattern separated with leaf-like edges, with thunder pattern on the bottom layer. Two characters " 亚㐭 " are inscribed near the dragon head on the inner bottom. It was acquired in 1958.

Preserved in The Palace Museum

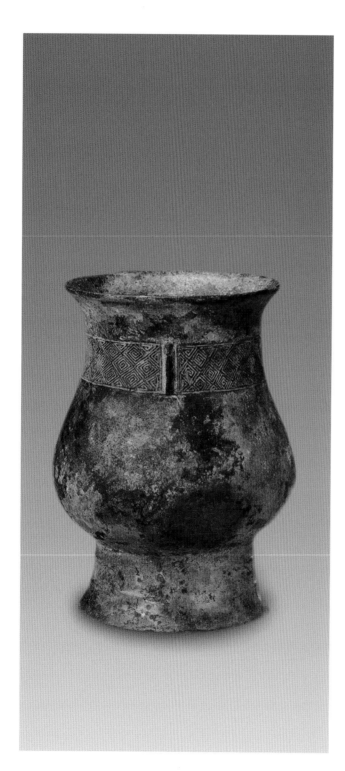

戉觯

商代晚期

青铜质

宽 9.5 厘米，通高 12 厘米，重 0.43 千克

Zhi with Characters Including ""

Late Shang Dynasty

Bronze

Width 9.5 cm/ Height 12 cm/ Weight 0.43 kg

侈口，束颈，垂腹，圈足较高。颈部饰斜向雷纹，中隔凸脊，圈足上饰两道弦纹。内底铸铭文 2 字。山东出土，1952 年国家文物局调拨。

故宫博物院藏

There is a wide mouth, a convergent neck, a drooping belly, and a long ring foot. The neck is decorated with thunder pattern with oblique angles. There is ridge in the middle of the vessel. There are two bands of bowstring pattern on the ring foot. The inner area of the bottom is inscribed 2 characters. It was unearthed in Shandong Province. The vessel was allocated from State Administration of Cultural Heritage in 1957.

Preserved in The Palace Museum

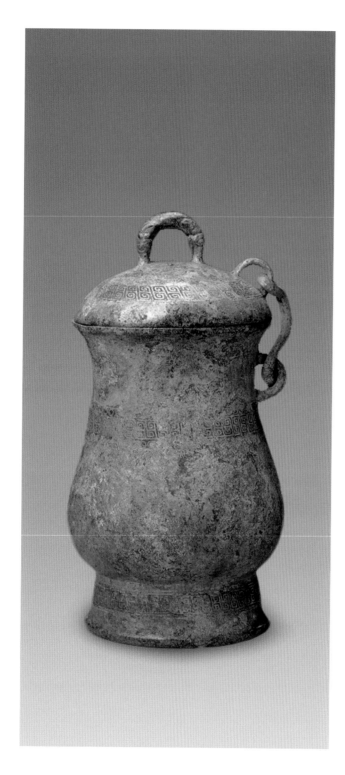

魚亚黾觯

商代晚期

青铜质

宽 9.7 厘米，通高 19.5 厘米，重 0.88 千克

Zhi with Characters Including "魚" and "黾"

Late Shang Dynasty

Bronze

Width 9.7 cm/ Height 19.5 cm/ Weight 0.88 kg

鼓腹，束颈，侈口，圈足。盖顶上有一双兽
组成的环钮，盖与器用链相连。盖、颈及足
均饰回纹一圈。盖内和器外底分别铸有铭文
"⊠"与"亚龟"。 1959 年收购。

故宫博物院藏

The vessel has a swelling belly, a convergent
neck, a wide mouth, and a ring foot. There is
a pedestal with a ring knob on the top of the
cover, and the cover is linked to the vessel
body with a chain. The cover, the neck and
the foot are all decorated with a rectangular
spiral pattern. On the inner side of the cover
and the outer surface of the bottom, there is an
inscription of 3 characters "⊠" and "亚龟". It
was acquired in 1959.

Preserved in The Palace Museum

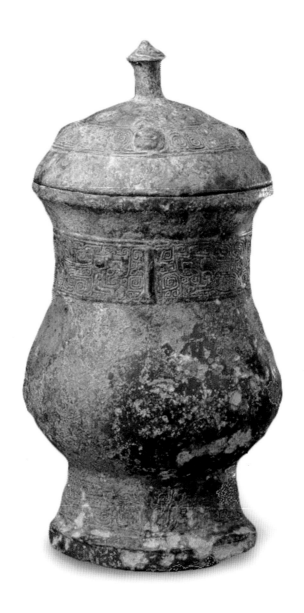

山妇觶

商代晚期

青铜质

口径 6 厘米，通高 17.5 厘米，重 0.66 千克

侈口，束颈，鼓腹，圈足，有盖。盖顶有一菌状钮，

饰雷纹；颈、足均有突棱，饰夔纹。器内有 2 字铭文。

1946 年入藏。

故宫博物院藏

Zhi with Characters "Shan Fu"

Late Shang Dynasty

Bronze

Mouth Diameter 6 cm/ Height 17.5 cm/ Weight 0.66 kg

The vessel has a wide mouth, a convergent neck, a drum abdomen, a ring foot, and a cover. The calibre of the vessel is shorter than the diameter of the belly. There is a mushroom-like knob on the top of the cover, which is decorated with thunder pattern. There is a protruding ridge on both the neck and the foot, decorated with Kui dragon pattern. There are 2 characters inscribed on the inside of the vessel. It was collected in 1946.

Preserved in The Palace Museum

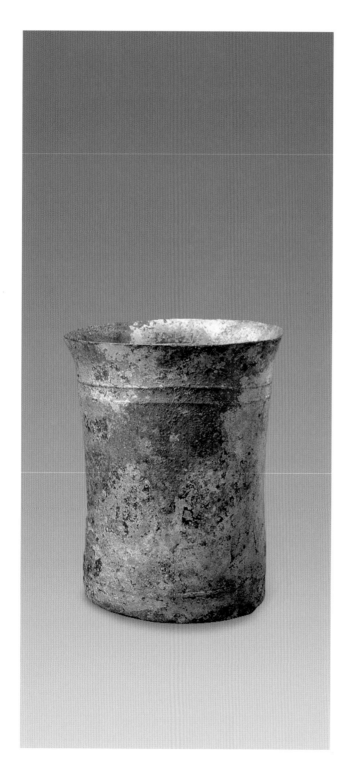

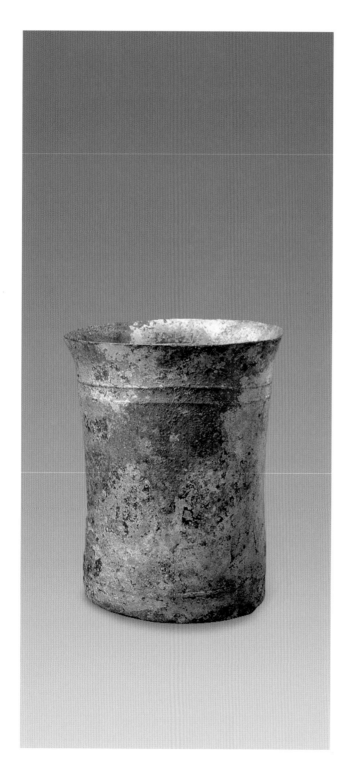觯

商代晚期

青铜质

宽 12.9 厘米，通高 15 厘米，重 0.98 千克

Zhi with Character ""

Late Shang Dynasty

Bronze

Width 12.9 cm/ Height 15 cm/ Weight 0.98 kg

体圆呈筒状，侈口，平底直壁，器壁向下
延伸形成圈足。通体只有颈部两道弦纹。
铭文"▨"字在器内壁上。1954 年收购。

　　　　　　　　　　　　　故宫博物院藏

The round and cannular drinking vessel has a
wide mouth, a flat bottom, and straight walls
extending downward and forming a ring foot.
There are two bands string pattern on the
neck. There is a character "▨" inscribed on
the inner wall. It was acquired in 1954.
Preserved in The Palace Museum

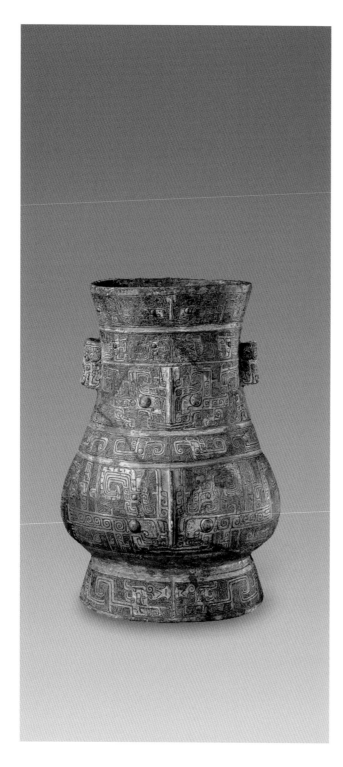

矢壶

商代晚期

青铜质

口径 19 厘米 ×14.5 厘米，宽 24.5 厘米，

高 34.6 厘米，重 6.49 千克

Bronze Pot with Character "Shi"

Late Shang Dynasty

Bronze

Mouth Diameter 19 cm×14.5 cm/ Width 24.5 cm/

Height 34.6 cm/ Weight 6.49 kg

形体扁圆，侈口，硕腹下垂，双贯耳，圈足。通体纹饰均以细密的回纹为地。从口沿至圈足共饰 6 层纹饰，分别间饰以兽面纹和夔纹，线条华丽流畅。双耳饰兽面纹。器底刻一 "矢" 字，因此为名。1946 年入藏。

故宫博物院藏

The pot has a flattened circular body, a wide flared mouth, a big and drooping belly, two tubular ears, and a ring foot. The whole pot is decorated with rectangular spiral pattern. From the mouth to the foot there are six layers of pattern. The interval of each layer is decorated with beast face pattern and Kui dragon pattern. The pattern is smooth and magnificent. The two ears are decorated with designs of beast face. On the bottom of the pot, a character "Shi" is carved, which gives this relic its name. The pot was collected in 1946.

Preserved in The Palace Museum

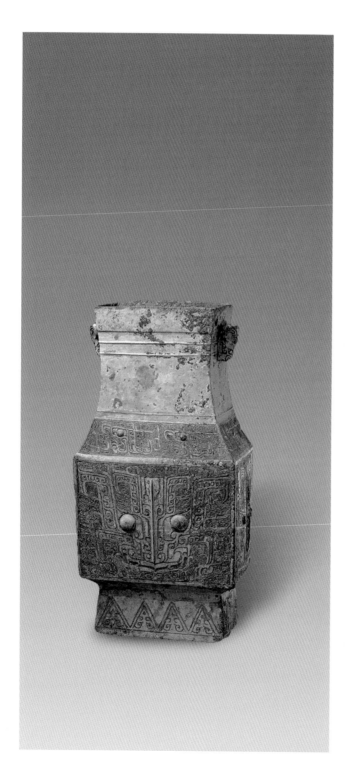

兽面纹方壶

商代晚期

青铜质

宽 19 厘米，高 34 厘米，重 3.7 千克

Square Bronze Pot with Animal Mask Pattern

Late Shang Dynasty

Bronze

Width 19 cm/ Height 34 cm/ Weight 3.7 kg

扁方形体，长颈，双贯耳，用以系绳提携，长方圈足。颈部饰两道弦纹，肩、腹部分别饰夔纹、兽面纹，均以细密的雷纹为地。兽面环睛突出，大嘴，很有神气。足部饰以蕉叶纹。1946 年入藏。

故宫博物院藏

The pot has a flattened and square body, a long neck, two tubular ears which are tied with strings for carrying purpose, and a rectangular ring foot. The neck is decorated with two belts of string patterns. The vessel's shoulder, and the belly are decorated respectively with Kui dragon pattern and design of beast face, both with delicate thunder patterns as ground-tint. The beast face has a vivid expression with protruding eyes and a big mouth. The foot is decorated with banana leaf pattern. The pot was collected in 1946.

Preserved in The Palace Museum

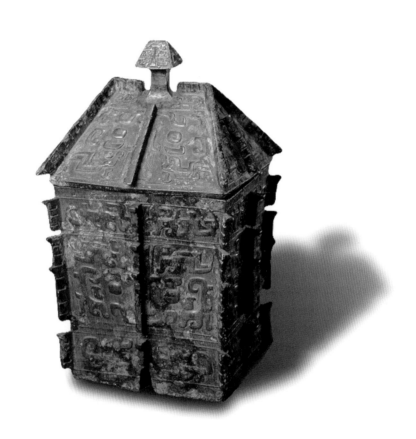

王生女齂方彝

商代晚期

青铜质

宽 18.6 厘米，通高 29.5 厘米，重 4.65 千克

Square Yi with Characters Including "齂"

Late Shang Dynasty

Bronze

Width 18.6 cm/ Height 29.5 cm/ Weight 4.65 kg

方体，深腹，直口，直壁。器腹向下延伸为足，盖呈屋顶形，顶上一钮，盖、腹、足均有八凸棱，足有四豁口。盖、腹、足均饰兽面纹。盖与器内均有铭文1行4字。吴秀源先生捐献。

故宫博物院藏

The vessel has a square body, a deep belly, a straight mouth, and straight walls. The foot is a part of the downward-stretching body of the vessel. The head cover is in a roof-like shape with a protruding knob on top of it. The cover the belly and foot are both decorated with eight convex ridges. The foot has four large openings. The cover and belly are also decorated with designs of beast face. The cover and inner part of the vessel both have an inscription of 4 characters in one line. The utensil was donated by Mr. Wu Xiuyuan.

Preserved in The Palace Museum

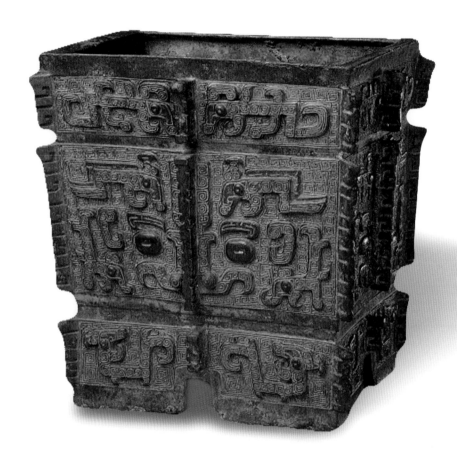

亚羲方彝

商代晚期

青铜质

宽 18.9 厘米，通高 17.9 厘米，重 3.34 千克

方体，深腹，平口沿，方圈足。足四面正中各有一"∩"形缺口，颈、腹、足上各有八条凸棱。颈及足均饰夔纹，夔呈爬行状，腹饰兽面纹，通身纹饰由三层花纹构成。器内底有铭文 2 字。清宫旧物（原藏颐和园）。

故宫博物院藏

Square Yi with Characters "Ya Xi"

Late Shang Dynasty

Bronze

Width 18.9 cm/ Height 17.9 cm/ Weight 3.34 kg

The vessel has a square body, a deep belly, a flattened mouth rim and a square ring foot. Each of the four sides of the foot has an inverted " ∩ " shape notch in the middle. The vessel neck, the belly and the foot are respectively decorated with 8 convex ridges. The neck and foot are both decorated with a creeping Kui dragon pattern. The belly is decorated with designs of beast face. The whole body is decorated with a three-layer pattern. There is an inscription of 2 characters on the inner bottom of the vessel. It was an antique from the imperial palace of the Qing Dynasty (originally preserved in the Summer Palace).

Preserved in The Palace Museum

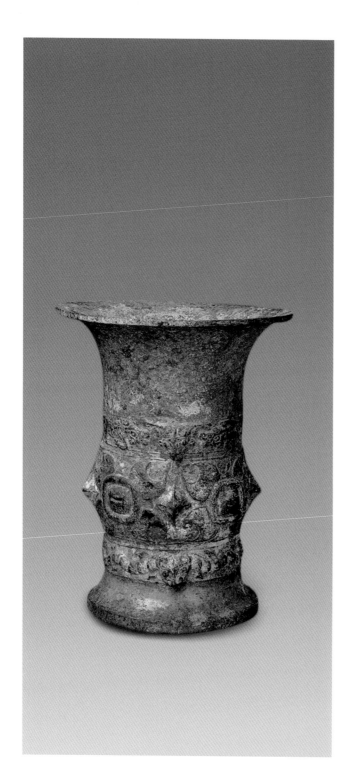

作尊彝尊

商代晚期

青铜质

宽 22.5 厘米，通高 27.6 厘米，重 3.35 千克

Zun with Characters "Zuo Zun Yi"

Late Shang Dynasty

Bronze

Width 22.5 cm/ Height 27.6 cm/ Weight 3.35 kg

圆体，侈口，深腹，圈足。腹部有三部分纹饰，上层饰牛纹，牛屈腿而卧；中层饰四条锥形凸棱，间饰四目纹，目纹四周有四瓣叶纹；下层饰单首双身龙纹。全部纹饰均采用半浮雕艺术手法，没有地纹衬托。器内底有铭文1行3字。1946年入藏。

故宫博物院藏

The vessel has a round body, a flare mouth, a deep belly, and a ring foot. The belly has three different decorations. The upper layer is decorated with cattle design with the cattle sitting down with its bending feet; the middle layer is decorated with four cone-like convex ridges, with eye-shaped pattern between each ridge surrounded by four-petal leaf design; the lower layer is decorated with a one-head two-body dragon pattern. All the decorations are achieved by the method of demirelief with no ground-tint. There is an inscription of 3 characters in one line on the bottom inside the vessel. The relic was collected in 1946.

Preserved in The Palace Museum

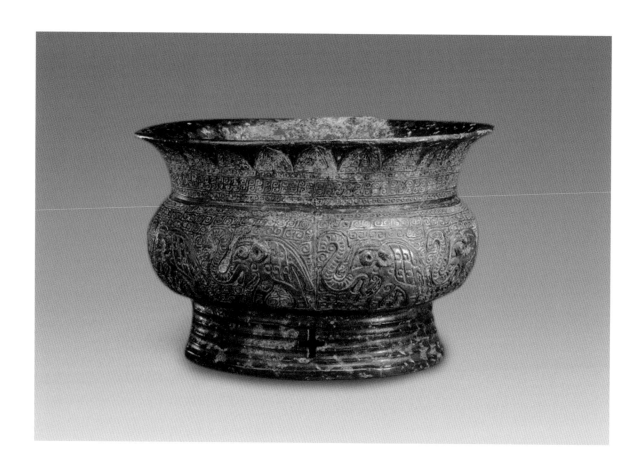

友尊

商代晚期

青铜质

口径 20.7 厘米，高 13.2 厘米，重 2.72 厘米

Zun with Character "You"

Late Shang Dynasty

Bronze

Mouth Diameter 20.7 cm/ Height 13.2 cm/ Weight 2.72 kg

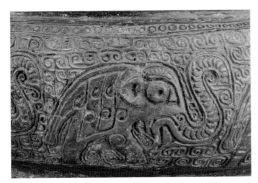

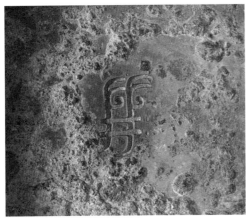

侈口，束颈圆腹，圈足。口沿下饰蕉叶纹、带状雷纹，二者间饰以联珠纹。腹部主要纹饰是九只长鼻高卷，相逐而行的大象，以云纹为地，象身再饰以线刻。圈足饰以横条沟脊纹，上有十字形孔。器内壁有一"友"字。传河南安阳出土，1960年北京市文化局调拨。

故宫博物院藏

The vessel has an flared mouth, a straight neck, a round belly, and a ring foot. Below the mouth rim there are decorations of banana leaf design and belt-like thunder pattern, with designs of a string of beads situating between the two. The belly is primarily decorated with nine elephants chasing each other with long and high-standing noses, with cloud pattern as ground-tint and line-carved reliefs of animal bodies. The ring foot is decorated with horizontal ridge pattern, also on the foot, there are 3 cross-like notchs. On the interior wall of the vessel there is a character " 友 ". It is said that the vessel was collected in Anyang City, Henan Province. The vessel was allocated from Beijing Municipal Bureau of Cultural in 1960.

Preserved in The Palace Museum

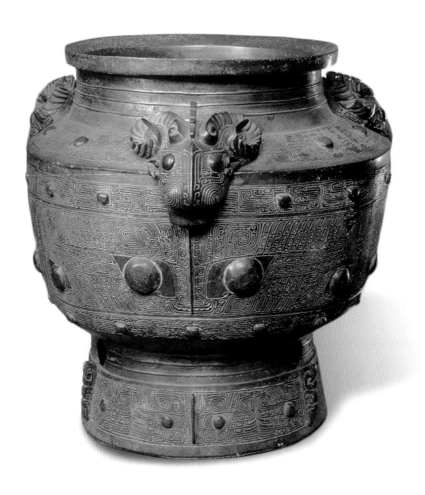

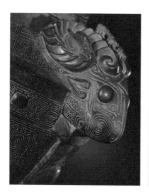
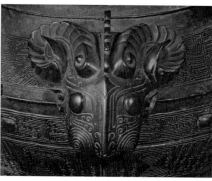
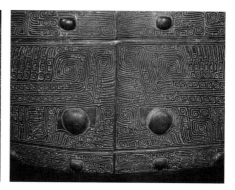

三羊尊

商代晚期

青铜质

口径 41.2 厘米，通高 52 厘米，重 51.3 千克

尊为大口广肩型，厚唇外折，细颈上有三道凸弦纹。肩部等距离地装饰三只高浮雕形式的卷角羊头，间以回形纹为地的目形纹饰。腹部较肥硕，纹饰更为华丽，在回形纹地上有三组兽面纹。圈足较高，上边有两条凸弦纹，中间有三个等距离的较大圆形孔，圈足的下部在回形纹地上饰了六组兽面纹。1956 年收购。

故宫博物院藏

Zun with Three Goats in Relief

Late Shang Dynasty

Bronze

Mouth Diameter 41.2 cm/ Height 52 cm/ Weight 51.3 kg

The vessel has a large mouth, a broad shoulder, and a thick lip which folds outward. There is a design of tree convex bowstrings on the thin neck. Designs of three high relief goat heads with curled horns are cast on the shoulder with equal space interval. Between the goat-head designs there is eye-shaped decoration with rectangular spiral pattern as ground-tint. The belly is relatively large with more foofaraw on it. There are three groups of beast face designs with rectangular spiral pattern as the ground-tint. The ring foot is tall, with two strips of convex string patterns on its upper section, three round-shaped holes with a fixed space interval in its middle section and six groups of beast face patterns in the lower section with rectangular spiral pattern as ground-tint. The relic was acquired in 1956.

Preserved in The Palace Museum

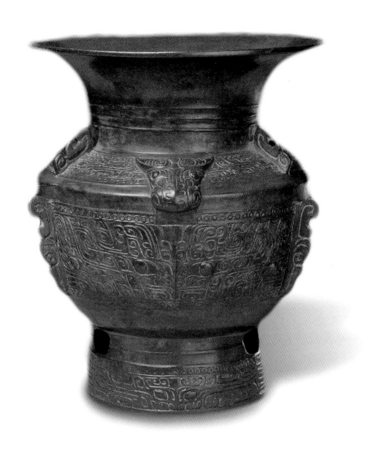

兽面纹尊

商代晚期

青铜质

口径 22.3 厘米，足径 13.4 厘米，宽 24 厘米，高 25.4 厘米，重 3.18 千克

Zun with Animal Mask Pattern

Late Shang Dynasty

Bronze

Mouth Diameter 22.3 cm/ Foot diameter 13.4 cm/ Width 24 cm/ Height 25.4 cm/ Weight 3.18 kg

大敞口，高圈足，足上有三个穿孔。颈饰三道弦纹，肩饰兽面纹，以联珠纹为边饰。肩上有三条云纹状棱脊，每两条脊之间浮雕一牛首，腹饰兽面纹，上下各饰一圈联珠纹。在肩部三条棱脊的下方，饰风格同样的三条棱脊。圈足也饰兽面纹，以联珠纹为边饰。清宫旧物（原藏颐和园）。

故宫博物院藏

The vessel has a large open mouth and a tall ring foot with three perforations on it. The neck is decorated with three belts of bowstrings, and the shoulder with beast face pattern edged with designs of a string of beads. On the shoulder, there are three strips of ridges in cloud-like pattern and there is a cattle head design in relief between two ridges. The belly is decorated with beast face designs, with a design of a string of beads on the upper and lower belly respectively. Below the three ridges on the shoulder there are another three ridges with the same style. The ring foot is also decorated with beast face designs edged with a string of bead pattern. The vessel was an antique from the imperial palace of the Qing Dynasty (originally kept in the Summer Palace)

Preserved in The Palace Museum

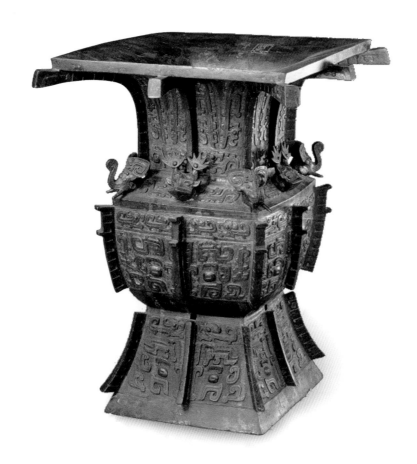

亚酰方尊

商代晚期

青铜质

宽 38 厘米，通高 45.5 厘米，重 21.5 千克

Square Zun with Characters Including "酰"

Late Shang Dynasty

Bronze

Width 38 cm/ Height 45.5 cm/ Weight 21.5 kg

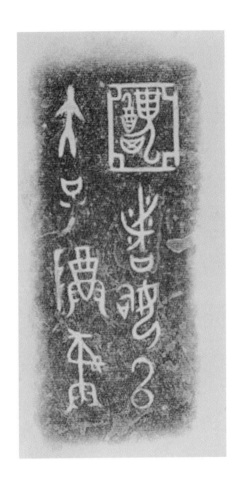

体呈正方形，侈口，鼓腹，高圈足。颈、腹、足均有纵向凸棱八条，肩上四角各有一立体象首，大耳，鼻上卷，双齿外露，两象首间饰一立体兽首。兽角向上呈花瓣状，颈部凸棱伸出口沿。颈饰夔纹，腹、足均饰兽面纹。铭文2行9字在口内壁上。清宫旧藏。

故宫博物院藏

The vessel has a square body, a flared mouth, a swelling belly, and a tall ring foot. There are eight vertical convex ridges on the neck, the belly, and the foot. There is a three-dimensional elephant head pattern with big ears, up rolling noses and exposed teeth on each of the four shoulders. Between two elephant head patterns there is a three-dimensional beast head pattern, with petal-like horn and protruding neck to the mouth of the vessel. The neck is decorated with Kui dragon pattern. There are beast face patterns on the belly and the foot. There is an inscription of 9 characters in 2 lines on the interior wall of the mouth of the vessel. The vessel was an antique from the imperial palace of the Qing Dynasty.

Preserved in The Palace Museum

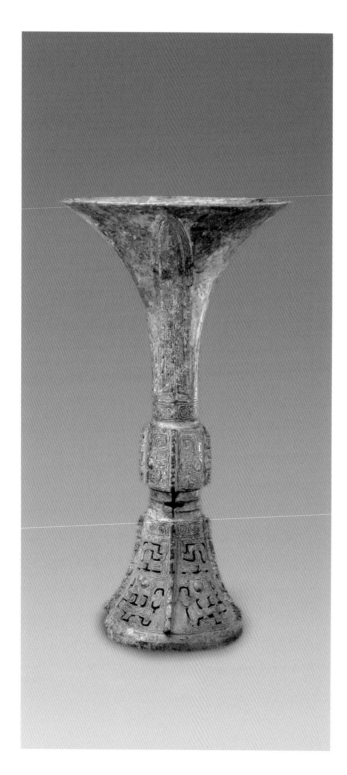

受觚

商代晚期

青铜质

宽 14.8 厘米，通高 26.4 厘米，重 0.93 千克

Gu with Character "Shou"

Late Shang Dynasty

Bronze

Width 14.8 cm/ Height 26.4 cm/ Weight 0.93 kg

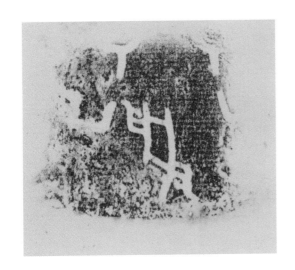

圆体，形似喇叭，侈口，细颈，高圈足，腰、足均有四凸棱。颈部饰蕉叶纹，腰饰兽面纹及二圈弦纹，足饰镂空透雕兽面纹。铭文一"受"字在足内壁上。1957 年收购。

故宫博物院藏

The vessel is round and shaped like a trumpet with a flared mouth, a thin neck, and a high ring foot. There are four convex ridges on both the waist and the ring foot. The neck is decorated with a plantain leaf-like pattern and beast face pattern and two circles of string patterns on the waist. The foot is decorated with beast face pattern in the style of bow hollowed-out openwork. There is an inscription of a character "Shou" on the wall of the foot. The vessel was acquired in 1957.

Preserved in The Palace Museum

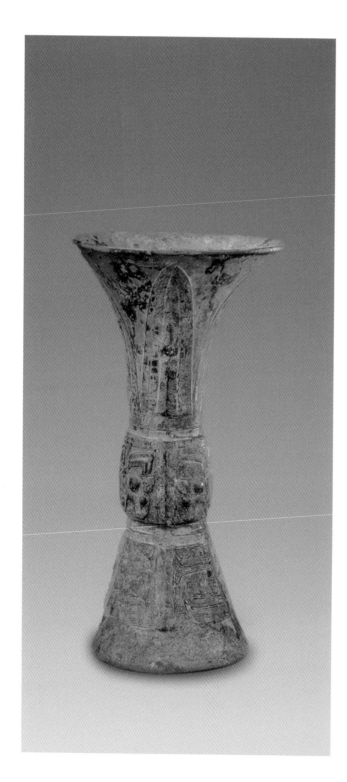

吴觚

商代晚期

青铜质

宽 12.9 厘米，通高 20.4 厘米，重 0.66 千克

Gu with Character "吴"

Late Shang Dynasty

Bronze

Width 12.9 cm/ Height 20.4 cm/ Weight 0.66 kg

体圆，形似喇叭，侈口，束腰，高圈足。颈
饰蕉叶纹，叶上有一凸脊，腰、足均饰兽面纹。
铭文一"吴"字在圈足内。1957 年收购。

故宫博物院藏

The vessel is round and similar in form to a
trumpet, with a flared mouth, a slender waist,
and a tall ring foot. The neck is decorated with
a plantain leaf-like pattern, with a ridge on the
leaf. There are beast face designs on both the
waist and the foot. There is an inscription of
a character " 吴 " on the inner area of the ring
foot. The vessel was acquired in 1957.
Preserved in The Palace Museum

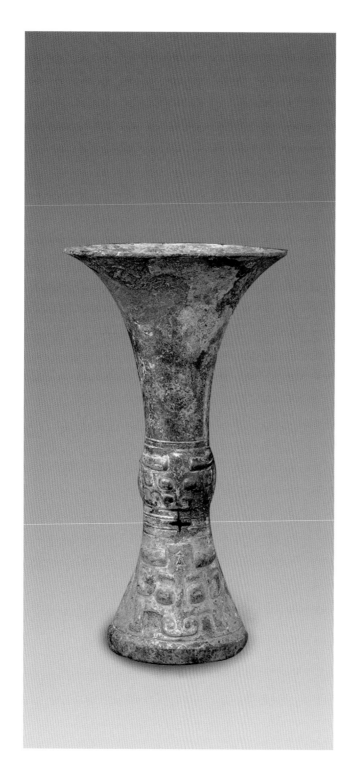

斧觚

商代晚期

青铜质

宽 15.5 厘米，通高 26.5 厘米，重 1.16 千克

Gu with Character "斧"

Late Shang Dynasty

Bronze

Width 15.5 cm/ Height 26.5 cm/ Weight 1.16 kg

体圆，形似喇叭，侈口，束腰，圈足。腰部前后各有一个十字孔，腰、足饰兽面纹。觚的铭文一般都在足内壁上，此觚的铭文"合"却在足外壁花纹上，这种现象比较少见。1957年收购。

故宫博物院藏

The vessel is round and similar in shape to a trumpet, with a flared mouth, a slender waist, and a ring foot. On the front and the back of the waist, there is one crisscross hole on each side of the waist. There are beast face designs on both the waist and the ring foot. The inscription of "Gu" is usually on the walls inside the foot, but the inscription "合" of this vessel is on the pattern of wall outside the foot, which is very rare. The vessel was acquired in 1957.

Preserved in The Palace Museum

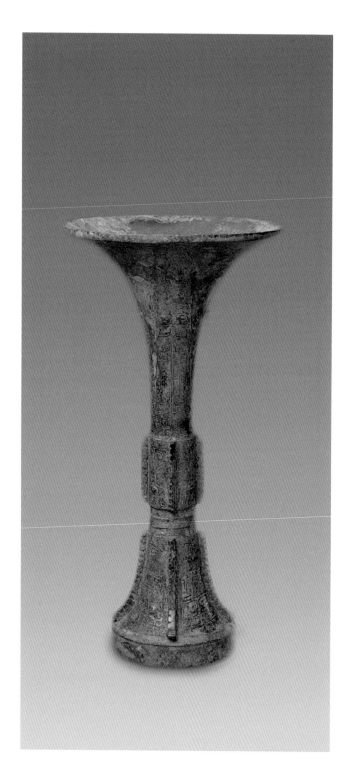

无终觚

商代晚期

青铜质

宽 17 厘米，通高 30.8 厘米，重 1.62 千克

Gu with Characters " Wu Zhong "

Late Shang Dynasty

Bronze

Width 17 cm/ Height 30.8 cm/ Weight 1.62 kg

整体呈喇叭形，长颈，侈口，束腰，圈足。腰、足各有四凸棱，颈饰蕉叶纹，叶上又饰兽面纹，腰及足饰兽面纹。方国名"无终"二字在足内壁上。"无终"二字是裘锡圭先生考释出的。1959 年北京市文化局调拨。

故宫博物院藏

This vessel is trumpet shaped with a long neck, a flared mouth, a slender waist, and a ring foot. There are four convex ridges on both the waist and the foot. The neck is decorated with a plantain leaf-like pattern, and a beast face pattern on the leaf. There are also beast face designs on both the waist and foot. There are two characters "Wu Zhong" on the inner wall of the foot which were interpreted-like by Mr. Qiu Xigui. The vessel was allocated from Beijing Municipal Bureau of Culture in 1959.

Preserved in The Palace Museum

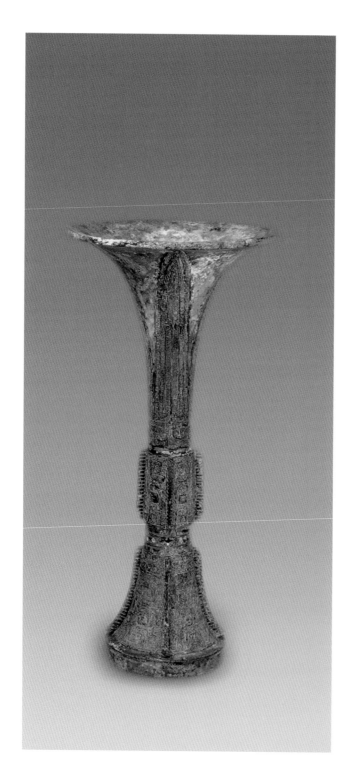

戬癸觚

商代晚期

青铜质

宽 16.3 厘米，通高 30.9 厘米，重 1.26 千克

Gu with Characters Including "戬"

Late Shang Dynasty

Bronze

Width 16.3 cm/ Height 30.9 cm/ Weight 1.26 kg

觚高体细，大口外侈，圈足，足下有一周狭边。颈饰伸长的蕉叶纹，腰、足均饰兽面纹。圈足内有 2 字铭文。1946 年入藏。

故宫博物院藏

The vessel has a high and thin body, a big flared mouth. There is a round of narrow margin under the ring foot. The neck is decorated with a long plantain leaf-like pattern. There are also beast face designs on both the waist and the foot. There is an inscription of 2 characters on the inner area of the ring foot. The vessel was collected in 1946.

Preserved in The Palace Museum

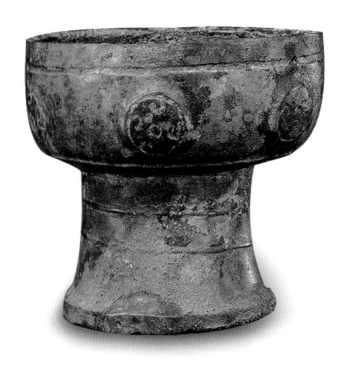

囗豆

商代晚期

青铜质

口径 12.1 厘米，通高 10.5 厘米，重 0.68 千克

Dou with Character " 囗 "

Late Shang Dynasty

Bronze

Mouth Diameter 12.1 cm/ Height 10.5 cm/ Weight 0.68 kg

圆体，直口，浅腹，直壁，高圈足。口下饰
凹弦纹一圈，腹饰涡纹，足饰弦纹二周。铭
文"▨"字在器内底上。1956 年收购。

故宫博物院藏

The round vessel has a straight mouth, a
shallow belly, straight walls, and a high ring
foot. There is a round of grooves bowstring
patterns under the mouth. The belly is decorated
with a vortex pattern. The foot is decorated with
two circles of bowstring patterns. There is an
inscription of "▨ " on the inner bottom of the
container. It was acquired in 1956.

Preserved in The Palace Museum

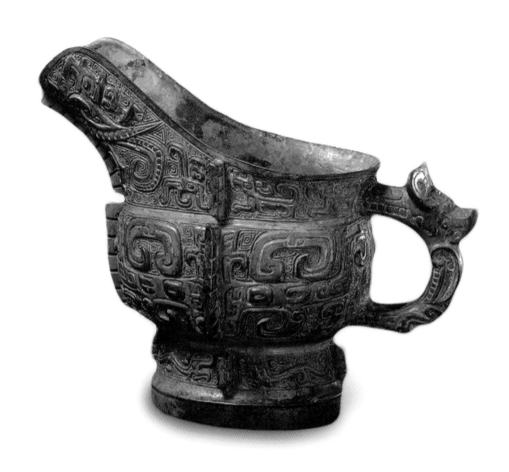

兽面纹兕觥

商代晚期

青铜质

宽 20 厘米，高 15 厘米，重 0.72 千克

Si Gong with Animal Mask Pattern

Late Shang Dynasty

Bronze

Width 20 cm/ Height 15 cm/ Weight 0.72 kg

椭圆形体，无盖，兽首鋬，高圈足。通体纹饰以多种形状的雷纹为衬地，流饰长尾鸟纹，口沿下饰夔纹，腹饰兽面纹，足饰一圈夔纹。流、口、足及腹均装饰有棱脊。1964 年 10 月收购。

故宫博物院藏

The vessel is oval in shape with no cover. There is an animal head handle and a tall ring foot. The whole body is decorated with thunder patterns in various styles as the ground-tint, and the spout is decorated with long-tailed bird pattern. The rim of the mouth is decorated with Kui dragon pattern, and the belly is decorated with beast face pattern, the ring foot with a circle of Kui dragon pattern. There are convex ridges on the spout, the mouth, and the belly. It was collected in October, 1964.

Preserved in The Palace Museum

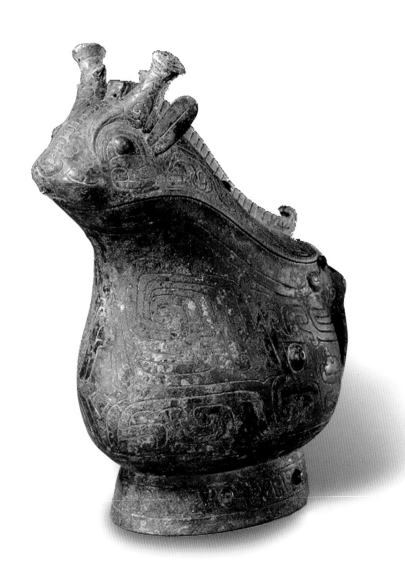

兽面纹兕觥

商代晚期

青铜质

宽 19.8 厘米，高 14.9 厘米，重 2.86 千克

通体呈兽形，有盖，兽首鋬，圈足。盖做成兽首状，双角间起棱脊，两侧饰夔纹。腹饰兽面纹，圈足饰以目雷纹。1955 年国家文物局调拨。

故宫博物院藏

Si Gong with Animal Mask Pattern

Late Shang Dynasty

Bronze

Width 19.8 cm/ Height 14.9 cm/ Weight 2.86 kg

The whole body is in the shape of a beast with a cover, an animal head handle, and a ring foot. The cover is in the shape of a beast head, and there is a convex ridge design between the two horns with Kui dragon pattern on both sides. The belly is decorated with beast face pattern, and the ring foot is decorated with thunder design. The vessel was allocated from State Administration of Cultural Heritage in 1955.

Preserved in The Palace Museum

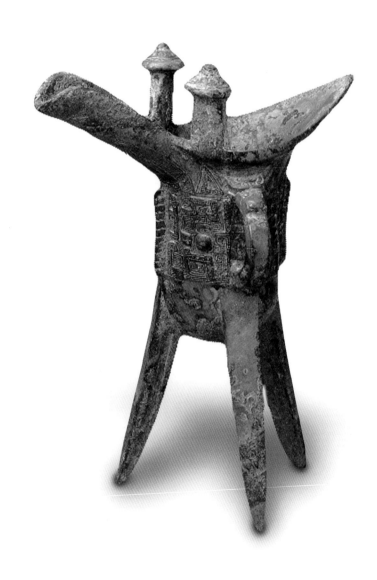

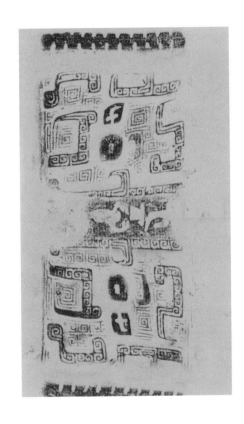

子工万爵

商代晚期

青铜质

宽 16 厘米，通高 21.1 厘米，重 0.76 千克

体圆，有流，有尾，三棱锥形足，口上有二菌形柱，腹上有一兽首鋬。口、流、尾下均饰蕉叶纹，腹饰兽面纹。铭文"子工万"3 字在鋬内。1953 年收购。

故宫博物院藏

Jue with Characters "Zi Gong Wan"

Shang Dynasty

Bronze

Width 16 cm/ Height 21.1 cm/ Weight 0.76 kg

The round vessel has a spout, a tail, prismatic tripodal feet, two fungus-shaped pillars on the mouth, and an animal head handle on the belly. There are decorations of plantain leaf-like patterns on the mouth, the spout, and the tail. The belly is decorated with beast face pattern. There is an inscription of 3 characters "Zi Gong Wan" on the inner side of the handle. It was acquired in 1953.

Preserved in The Palace Museum

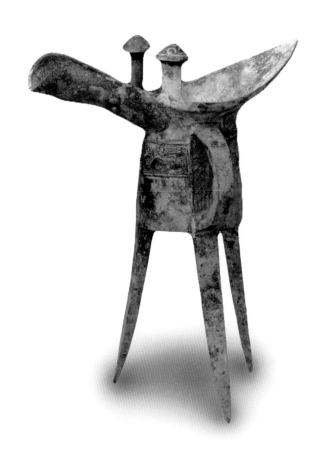

何宄父癸爵

商代晚期

青铜质

宽 16.6 厘米，通高 19.9 厘米，重 0.58 千克

Jue with Characters Including " 宄 "

Late Shang Dynasty

Bronze

Width 16.6 cm/ Height 19.9 cm/ Weight 0.58 kg

圆腹，平底，有流，有尾，口上有二菌形柱，腹上有一鋬，腹下有三棱锥形足。柱顶饰涡纹，腹饰夔纹一周。鋬内铸铭文4字"何歖父癸"。1958年收购。

故宫博物院藏

The vessel has a round belly and a flat bottom, with a spout and a tail. There are two fungus-shaped pillars on the mouth, a handle on the belly, and three prismatic tripodal feet under the belly. The top of the pillar is decorated with a vortex pattern, and a circle of Kui dragon designs on the belly. On the inner side of the handle, there is an inscription of 4 characters. It was acquired in 1958.

Preserved in The Palace Museum

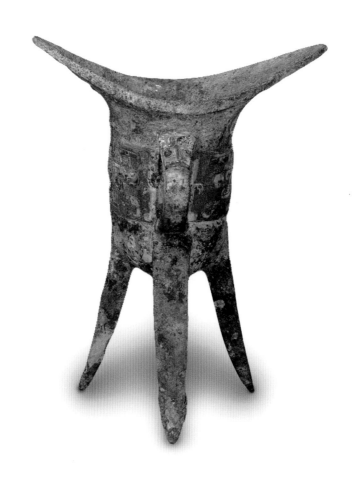

父己角

商代晚期

青铜质

宽 16.5 厘米，通高 20.5 厘米，重 1 千克

Jiao with Characters "Fu Yi"

Late Shang Dynasty

Bronze

Width 16.5 cm/ Height 20.5 cm/ Weight 1 kg

圆体，深腹，侈口，双尾。腹上一兽首鋬，

三棱锥形足。腹饰兽面纹。铭文"父已"2字

在鋬内。1960 年收购。

故宫博物院藏

The round vessel has a deep belly, a large flared

mouth, and a double-tail. There is an animal

head handle on the belly, and tripodal feet.

The belly is decorated with beast face pattern.

On the inner side of the handle, there is an

inscription of 2 characters "Fu" and "Yi". It was

acquired in 1960.

Preserved in The Palace Museum

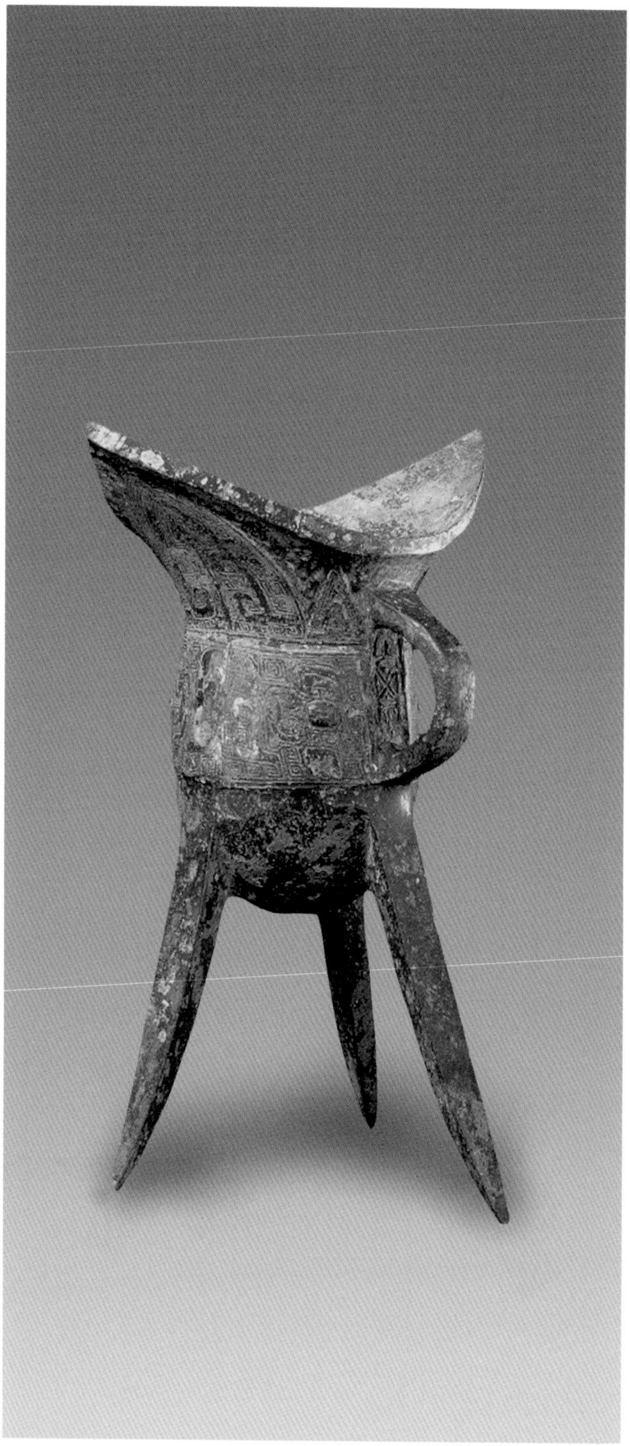

▨ 角

商代晚期

青铜质

宽 16.5 厘米，通高 20.8 厘米，重 0.84 千克

Jiao with Character "▨"

Late Shang Dynasty

Bronze

Width 16.5 cm/ Height 20.8 cm/ Weight 0.84 kg

圆腹，圜底，束颈，侈口，双角，腹侧有一
鋬，腹下有三棱锥形足。角下、颈部饰蕉叶
纹，腹部饰兽面纹。铭文一"▨"字在鋬内。
1946 年入藏。

故宫博物院藏

The vessel has a round belly, a round bottom,
a slender neck, a large flared mouth, and two
horns. There is a handle on one side of the belly,
and tripodal feet under the belly. Both the lower
horn and the neck are decorated with plantain
leaf-like patterns. The belly is decorated with
beast face pattern. There is an inscription of a
character "▨" on the inner side of the handle.
It was collected in 1946.

Preserved in The Palace Museum

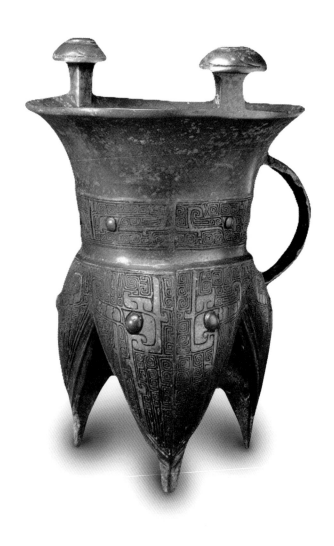

兽面纹斝

商代晚期

青铜质

宽 27.5 厘米，通高 34 厘米，重 3.58 千克

圆形体，侈口，上有二菌形柱，束腰，腹上有一鋬，三袋状足。柱顶饰涡纹，腹足饰兽面纹。1954 年国家文物局调拨。

故宫博物院藏

Jia with Animal Mask Pattern

Late Shang Dynasty

Width 27.5 cm/ Height 34 cm/ Weight 3.58 kg

The round vessel has a large flared mouth on which there are two mushroom-shaped columns and a wasp waist. There is a handle on the belly, bag-like tripodal pointed legs. The top of the columns is decorated with vortex pattern, and the belly and the legs are decorated with beast face pattern. The vessel was allocated from State Administration of Cultural Heritage in 1954.

Preserved in The Palace Museum

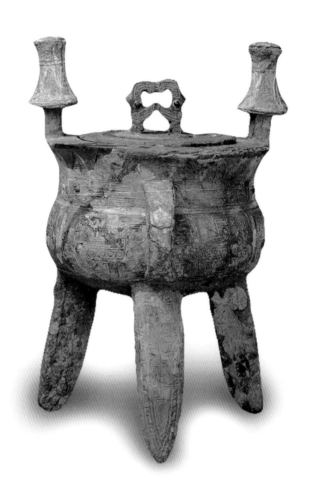

正斝

商代晚期

青铜质

宽 19 厘米，通高 26.1 厘米，重 2.66 千克

Jia with Character "Zheng"

Late Shang Dynasty

Bronze

Width 19 cm/ Height 26.1 cm/ Weight 2.66 kg

圆体，束颈，三棱形足，素扁錾，有盖，双伞形柱。柱顶饰涡纹，下饰弦纹、蕉叶纹及回纹，颈饰蕉叶纹及兽面纹，腹饰兽面纹，足饰蕉叶兽面纹。盖上一钮，钮上双鸟相背而立，尖嘴，大冠，圆睛突出，钮周围饰目雷纹一圈。口沿处有铭文"正"字。1958年上海文物管理委员会调拨。

故宫博物院藏

The vessel is supported by prismatic triangular legs. It has a round body and a slender neck, a plain flat handle, and a cover with twin umbrella-like columns. The top of the columns is decorated with vortex pattern. The lower part of the columns with bowstring pattern, banana leaf pattern, and rectangular spiral pattern (a kind of pattern which looks like the Chinese character "回"). The neck is decorated with banana leaf pattern and animal mask pattern, the belly with beast face pattern, the legs with banana leaf pattern and beast face pattern. There is a knob on the cover and the knob is decorated with two birds standing back to back with a sharp peak, big crest, bulging out eyes. The areas around the knob are decorated with eye-like and thunder pattern. There is an inscription of one character "Zheng" on the rim of the mouth. The vessel was allocated from Shanghai Administration of Committee of Cultural Relice in 1958.

Preserved in The Palace Museum

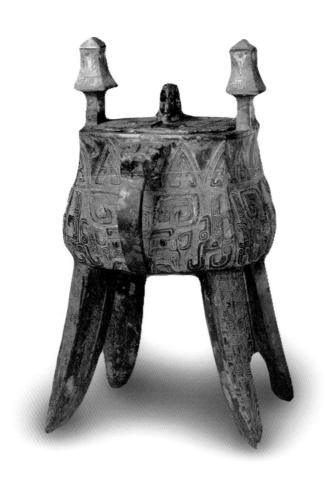

册方斝

商代晚期

青铜质

宽 16.2 厘米，通高 28.5 厘米，重 3.12 千克

Jia with Characters "Ce Fang"

Late Shang Dynasty

Bronze

Width 16.2 cm/ Height 28.5 cm/ Weight 3.12 kg

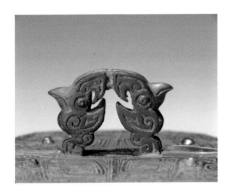

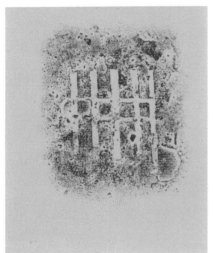

体方，有盖，四足。盖饰兽面纹，正中以两立鸟为钮。口沿与柱帽上均饰三角仰叶纹。腹部饰凸起的兽面纹，兽面两侧有倒夔纹，下以云雷纹为地。鋬上雕饰兽首。四足饰云雷纹、夔纹，呈蕉叶形。通体绿锈，甚为美观。斝的铭文大都在鋬下，此斝只在器内底上铭有一个"册"字。饮酒器。1957 年国家文物局调拨。

故宫博物院藏

The vessel has a square body, four legs, and a cover. The cover is decorated with beast face pattern with a knob shaped like two standing birds in the center of the cover. The rim of the mouth and the cap of the column are decorated with triangle leaf veins extending upward. The belly is decorated with animal mask patterns, the two sides of which there are reversed Kui dragon patterns with cloud and thunder pattern as the ground-tint. The handle is decorated with a sculpture in the shape of an animal head. The four legs are decorated with cloud and thunder pattern, Kui dragon pattern shaped like banana leaves. The whole body is in the color of patina looking extremely attractive. The majority of the inscription of a character "Ce" is beneath the handle. This "Jia", however, only has one character written as "Ce" on the inner side of the bottom. This served as a wine vessel in Late Shang Dynasty. The vessel was allocated from State Administration of Cultural Heritage in 1957.
Preserved in The Palace Museum

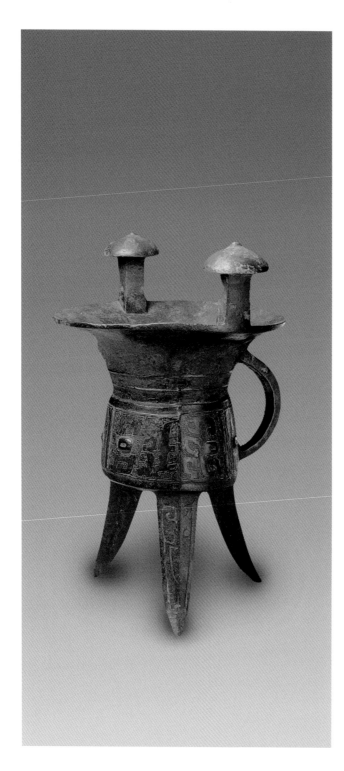

亚骖䍩

商代晚期

青铜质

宽 23.9 厘米，通高 30 厘米，重 2.18 千克

Jia with Characters Including "䍩"

Late Shang Dynasty

Bronze

Width 23.9 cm/ Height 30 cm/ Weight 2.18 kg

圆体，侈口，深腹，平底。口上有二菌形柱，腹侧有一素鋬，三尖足外侈。颈饰弦纹二圈，腹饰兽面纹。铭文"亚醜"2字在口上。清宫旧藏。

故宫博物院藏

The vessel has a round body, a flared mouth, a deep belly, and a flat bottom. There are two columns shaped like a mushroom on the mouth, and there is a plain handle on one side of the vessel. The body of the vessel is supported by sharp tripodal legs extending outward. The neck is decorated with two circles of bowstring patterns while the belly with animal mask pattern. This served as a wine vessel in Late Shang Dynasty. The inscription of 2 characters is on the mouth. It was an antique from the imperial palace of the Qing Dynasty.

Preserved in The Palace Museum

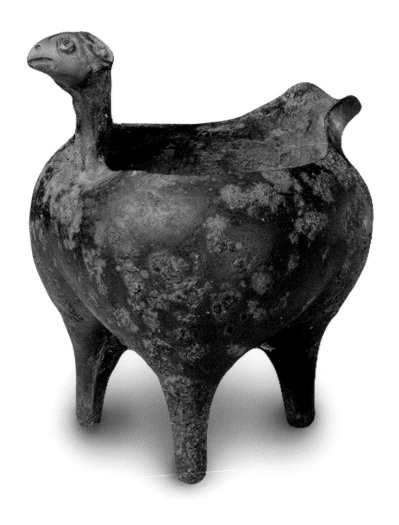

鸟首柄器

商代晚期

青铜质

宽 16.5 厘米，通高 17.3 厘米，重 1 千克

圆腹，敛口，口上有流和一鸟首柄，腹下有三足。器体光素无纹。鸟首柄器造型看似简单，但构思、设计很巧妙。整体呈鸟状，柄为颈，流为尾，像一只大鸟昂首站立，目视前方。1960 年北京市文化局调拨。

故宫博物院藏

Utensil with a Bird-head Shaped Handle

Late Shang Dynasty

Bronze

Width 16.5 cm/ Height 17.3 cm/ Weight 1 kg

The utensil has a folding rim and a round belly supported by tripodal legs under the belly. It has a small mouth with a spout and a handle shaped like a bird's head. The utensil is plain and has no patterns. The design of the bird head handle is ingenious and elaborate though it looks simple. The whole utensil is in the shape of a bird with the bird's neck as the handle and the bird's tail as the spout; thus it resembles a large bird that stands still and looks forward. The vessel was allocated from State Administration of Cultural Heritage in 1960.

Preserved in The Palace Museum

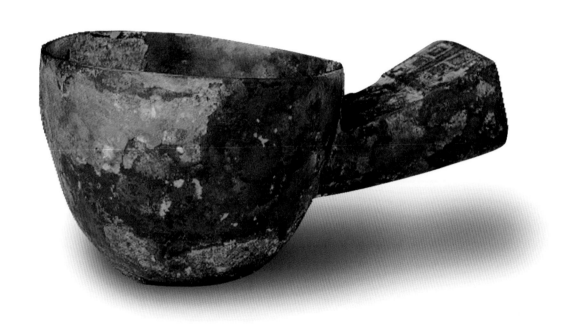

册勺

商代晚期

青铜质

长 12.3 厘米，宽 7.8 厘米，通高 5.2 厘米，重 0.32 千克

Ladle with Character "册"

Late Shang Dynasty

Bronze

Length 12.3 cm/ Width 7.18 cm/ Height 5.2 cm/ Weight 0.32 kg

直口，圆腹，圜底，腹侧有一柄。柄中空，呈半圆筒状，一端粗，一端细，上有二圆孔。铭文"田"字在柄上。1959 年北京市文化局调拨。

故宫博物院藏

The ladle has a straight mouth, a round belly, and a ring bottom with a handle on one side of the belly. The handle is hollow and in the shape of half cylinder with one end being small and the other end being large. There are two holes on the handle, and the inscription of the character "田" is on the handle. The ladle was allocated from the Beijing Municipal Bareau of Cultural in 1959.

Preserved in The Palace Museum

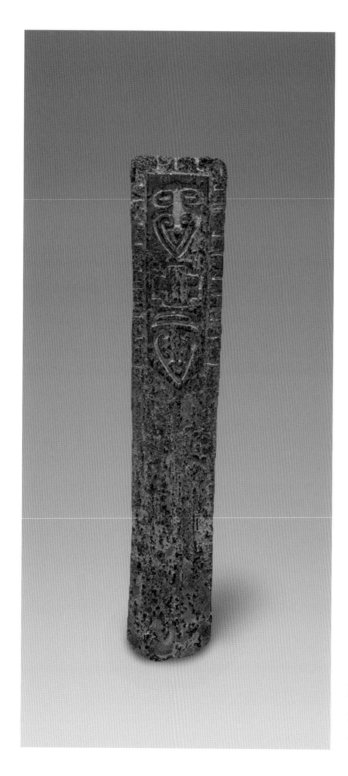

亚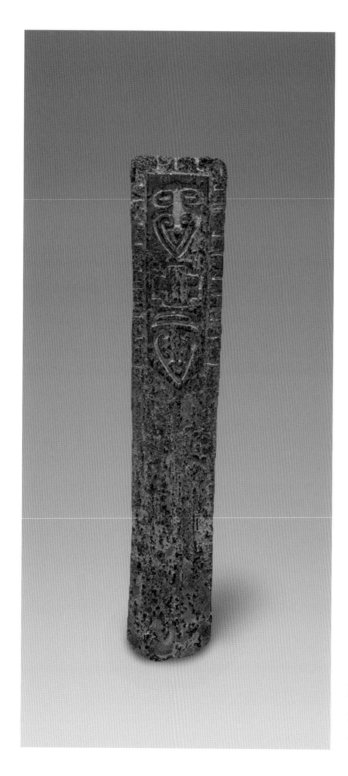匕

商代晚期

青铜质

宽 3.8 厘米，通高 20.2 厘米，重 0.14 千克

Bi with Characters Including "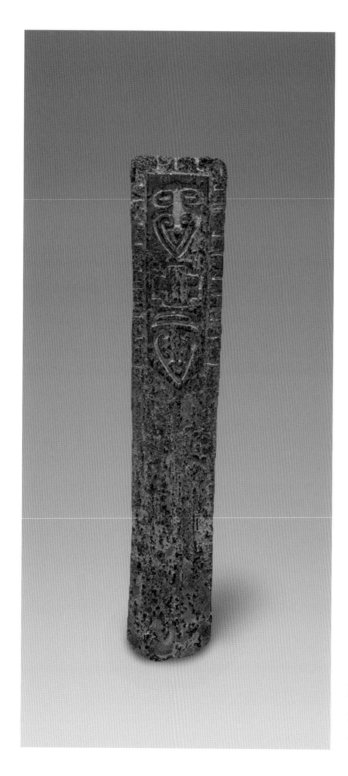"

Late Shang Dynasty

Bronze

Width 3.8 cm/ Height 20.2 cm/ Weight 0.14 kg

边棱由后往前渐趋隐没，上有短线纹。器体上部有 1 行 2 字铭文，商代的匕有文字者较少见。匕是挹取饭食或牲肉的器具，多与鼎、鬲相伴出土。1957 年收购。

故宫博物院藏

The vessel is an ancient type of spoon. Its edge is gradually shaded from the posterior to the anterior, with short line patterns. There is an inscription of 2 characters in one line on the upper part of the vessel. The vessel was utilized for ladling food and is commonly excavated together with tripod caldrons (ancient cooking vessels) and Li (ancient cooking tripods with hollow legs). It was rare to have an inscriptions on a Bi in the Shang Dynasty. It was acquired in 1957.

Preserved in The Palace Museum

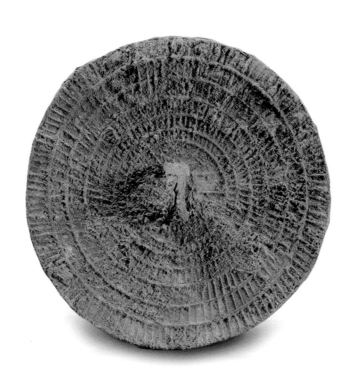

同心圆纹镜

商代晚期

铜质

直径 11.8 厘米

Mirror with Design of Concentric Circles

Late Shang Dynasty

Copper

Diameter 11.8 cm

弓形钮，以镜钮为圆心，饰同心圆纹，六圆环间密布竖直短线，形成由内向外辐射状光芒。此镜较薄，纹饰简练，是目前出土的较早铜镜之一。1976 年河南安阳殷墟妇好墓出土。

中国社会科学院考古研究所藏

The mirror has an arch-like knob at its center. The mirror is decorated with six concentric circles filled with short straight lines radiating outwards. Being thin and concise in design with decorative patterns, the mirror is one of the earlier bronze mirrors excavated at present. It was excavated in the Tomb of Fuhao in Anyang City, Henan Province, in 1976.

Preserved in Institute of Archaeology, Chinese Academy of Social Sciences

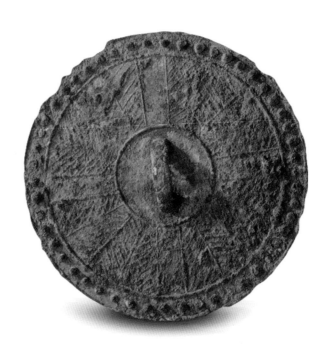

叶脉纹镜

商代晚期

铜质

直径 12.5 厘米

Mirror with Design of Leaf Veins

Late Shang Dynasty

Copper

Diameter 12.5 cm

弓形钮,镜背饰凸弦纹三周,一周平素无纹饰。二周四出平行双线把镜纹分为四区,每区由放射直线、斜线组成排列有序、茎脉分明的两片树叶形,相对两区纹饰相同。外侧整齐排列乳钉一周。1976年河南安阳殷墟妇好墓出土。

中国社会科学院考古研究所藏

The mirror has an arch-like knob. The rear of the mirror is decorated with three circles of convex string patterns. The first circle is plain and lacks decorative patterns. In the second circle, the mirror is divided by four pairs of parallel lines into quarters. Each quarter contains radiating straight lines, with which diagonal lines intersect, thus forming a leaf-like pattern. This pattern resembles two leaves with orderly patterns and apparent veins. These two leaves are reflected to form four quarters. The third circle is lined up with papillae. It was excavated in the Tomb of Fuhao in Anyang City, Henan Province, in 1976.

Preserved in Institute of Archaeology, Chinese Academy of Social Sciences

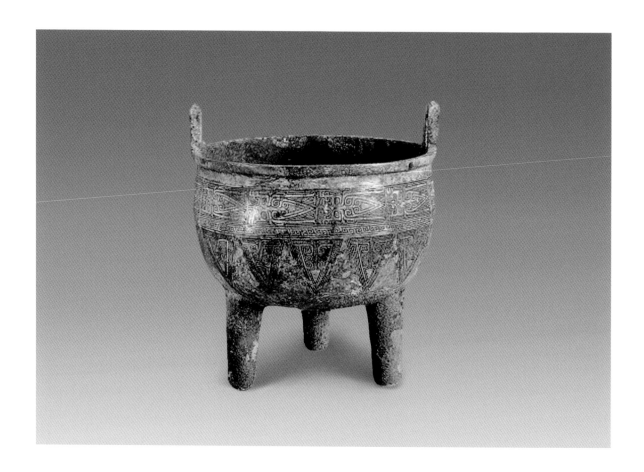

青铜蝉纹鼎

商

青铜质

口径 20 厘米，高 22.3 厘米

Bronze Tripod with Cicada Pattern

Shang Dynasty

Bronze

Mouth Diameter 20 cm/ Height 22.3 cm

造型浑圆厚重，但形体娇小，图案疏密得当，层次分明，装饰风格透出浓郁的现实生活气息。内壁底面上铸有家族的徽号。

北京大学赛克勒考古与艺术博物馆藏

The design of the tripod is round and massive but small in size. The patterns on it are appropriately spaced and properly structured. The decor reveals a rich breath of the real life. On the bottom inside the tripod, there is the family emblem.

Preserved in Arthur M. Sackler Museum of Art and Archaeology at Peking University

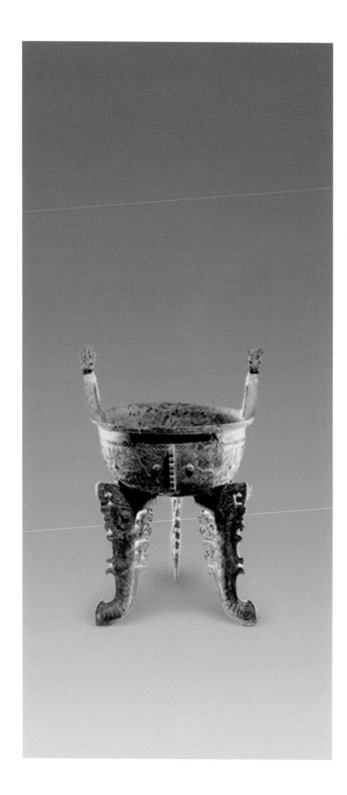

龙虎耳青铜扁足鼎

商

青铜质

口径 39.3 厘米，通高 64 厘米

Flat-legged Bronze Tripod with Dragon and Tiger Shaped Handles

Shang Dynasty

Bronze

Mouth Diameter 39.3 cm/ Height 64 cm

造型和装饰别致,在已发现的扁足青铜鼎中,此为形制最巨者。炊具。江西省新干县大洋洲商代大墓出土。

江西省博物馆藏

The tripod, with a unique design and decor, is the most massive one among those flat-legged bronze tripods that have been discovered. It was used as a cooking vessel. It was unearthed from the Shang Tomb in Dayangzhou, Xingan County, Jiangxi Province.

Preserved in Jiangxi Provincial Museum

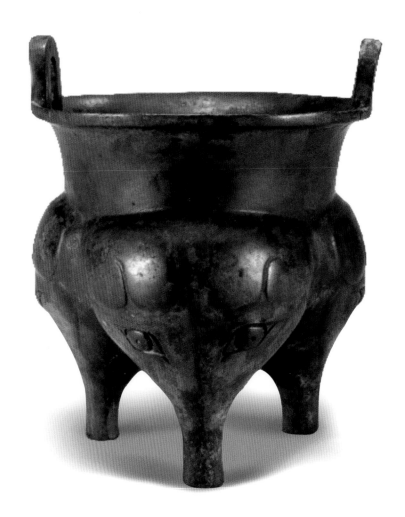

兽面纹鬲

商

青铜质

宽 16.5 厘米，高 16.8 厘米

体圆，束颈，侈口，双立耳，三足，足饰兽面纹。

鬲属食器。

故宫博物院藏

Li with Animal Mask Pattern

Shang Dynasty

Bronze

Width 16.5 cm/ Height 16.8 cm

This cooking vessel has a round body, a narrowed neck, a large mouth, two prick ears, and three legs on which there are beast face designs.

Preserved in The Palace Museum

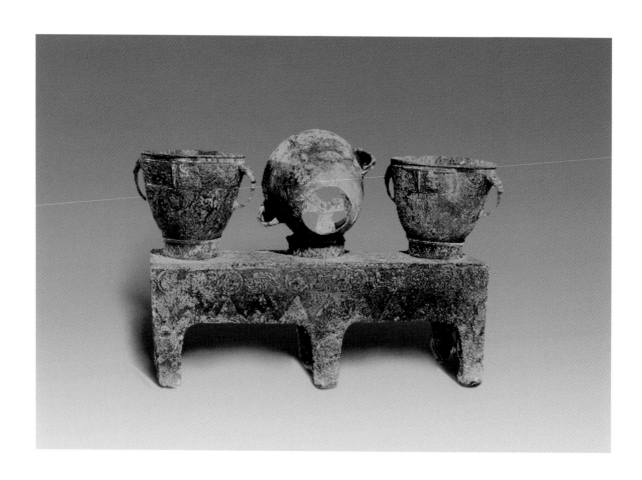

妇好三联甗

商（前 16 世纪—前 11 世纪）

青铜质

通长 103.7 厘米，通高 68 厘米，重 138.2 千克

Triple Yan with Characters "Fuhao"

Shang Dynasty (16th Century B.C.–11st Century B.C.)

Bronze

Length 103.7 cm/ Height 68 cm/ Weight 138.2 kg

本身为甑、鬲组成的复合炊具，此件系 3 个甗的鬲合为一体，甑则仍然是 3 个个体，形成一鬲加三甑的复合炊具格局。3 个甑口径 32.6~33 厘米，高 26.2~26.6 厘米，大小相若而略有差异。构思与造型不凡，装饰丰富而和谐，充分反映商代中期青铜铸造技术和装饰艺术所达到的水平。中间鬲口的内壁、甑的内壁及两耳下的外壁，都有"妇好"二字铭文。该器是名副其实的青铜重器，被列为国宝级的文物。河南省安阳市殷墟妇好墓出土。

中国社会科学院考古研究所藏

This steaming cooker is composed of Zeng steamer caldron and Li cooking vessel. It is a compound cooking vessel with three Li in a set and three Zeng. The Mouth Diameter of the three Zeng is 32.6−33 cm, and the height is 26.2−26.6 cm, and they have a similar yet slightly different size. The decoration of the vessel is rich and in harmony with its extraordinary ideas and modeling, which fully demonstrates high level of casting technology and decorative art of bronze ware in Mid-Shang Dynasty. The inner wall at the center of the Li's mouth and Zeng, and the outer wall below the two ears are engraved with characters "Fu Hao". It is listed as a national level cultural treasure. It was unearthed in Fuhao Tomb of Yin Ruins, Anyang City, Henan Province.

Preserved in The Institute of Archaeology, Chinese Academy of Social Science

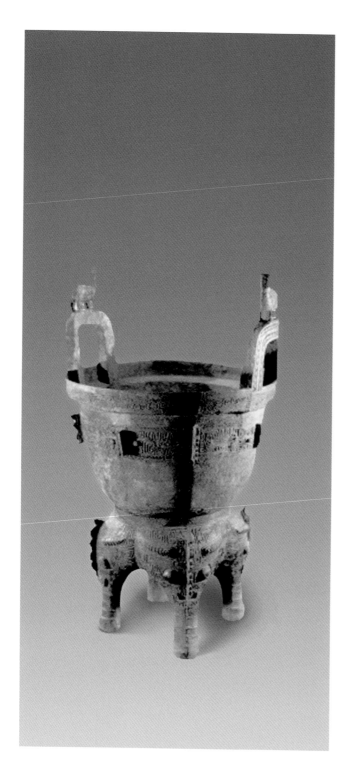

立鹿耳四足青铜甗

商（前 16 世纪—前 11 世纪）

青铜质

上口径 61.2 厘米，通高 105 厘米

Four-legged Bronze Yan with Standing Deer Handles

Shang Dynasty (16th Century B.C.–11st Century B.C.)

Bronze

Upper Diameter 61.2 cm/ Height 105 cm

甗为上甑下鬲的合体。此件下部鬲有四条长足，这在已发现的青铜甗中实属凤毛麟角，而且通高达一米以上，伟形巨制，使之成为目前所知形制最大的青铜甗。江西新干县大洋洲商代大墓出土。

江西省博物馆藏

The bronze Yan is a combination of Zeng steamer caldron (upper part) and Li cooking vessel (lower part). The lower part of this vessel has four long legs, which is quite rare among the bronze Yan vessels. And this great work of art is more than a meter in height, which is the largest among the bronze Yan. It was unearthed in the tomb of the Shang Dynasty of Dayangzhou Town, Xingan County, Jiangxi Province.

Preserved in Jiangxi Provincial Museum

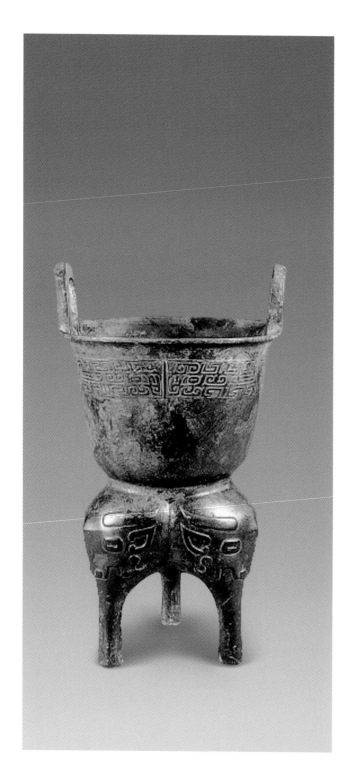

青铜甗

商（前 13 世纪—前 11 世纪）

青铜质

口径 20.9 厘米，高 35.4 厘米

Bronze Yan

Shang Dynasty (13rd Century B.C.–11st Century B.C.)

Bronze

Mouth Diameter 20.9 cm/ Height 35.4 cm

商代的铜甗是新石器时代晚期陶甗的继承与发展，在功能上仍然是煮水蒸食的蒸锅，形态上也是上甑下鬲并连为一体的组合。但由于青铜铸造业的发达及社会审美趣味的变化，商代铜甗的造型更加规范，装饰也更加繁杂。此件器身匀称，器表光洁。上部内壁有族徽符号。

北京大学赛克勒考古与艺术博物馆藏

The bronze Yan steaming cooker in the Shang Dynasty, inherited and developed from the pottery Yan in late Neolithic Age. Its function is still a combination of steaming food on the upper part and cooking food by boiling water in the lower part. In the structure, it is a combination of Zeng steamer caldron (upper part) and Li cooking vessel (lower part). However, with the development of foundry industry of bronze ware and the changes of aesthetic interest of the society, the shapes of bronze are Yan in the Shang Dynasty were more standardized, and the decorations were more elaborate and rich. This bronze Yan is well-shaped with smooth surfaces. The inner walls of the upper part are carved with the symbol of the emblem for a clan.

Preserved in Arthur M. Sackler Museum of Art and Archaeology at Peking University

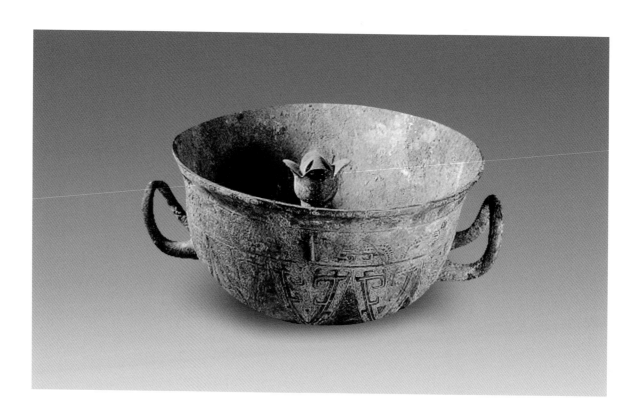

青铜气柱甑

商（前 16 世纪—前 11 世纪）

青铜质

口径 31 厘米，高 15.6 厘米

柱：高 13.1 厘米

Bronze Zeng with a Steam Pillar

Shang Dynasty (16th Century B.C.–11st Century B.C.)

Bronze

Mouth Diameter 31 cm/ Height 15.6 cm

Column: Height 13.1 cm

外形似一敞口深腹盆，腹侧有一对附耳，底内中部有一个中空透底的圆柱，柱头为四片立体花瓣形，包裹一中心突起的花蕾，花蕾表面有四个柳叶形的镂孔。腹内壁上有"好"字铭文。此件系三千多年前的蒸汽铜锅，且为迄今发现最早也是唯一的一件商代气锅。河南省安阳市殷墟妇好墓出土。

河南博物院藏

The vessel has a wide mouth, deep belly and a pair of attached handles. In the center of the inner bottom, there is a hollow column that is penetrable to the bottom. The head of the column is in tri-dimensional petal shape with four petals that wraps a protuberant as a bud. On the surface of the bud, there are four holes carved in willow leaf-shape. On the inner wall of the belly, there is an inscription of the character "hao". This vessel is a bronze steam pot, and it is the earliest and the only one among all the known steam pots in the Shang Dynasty. It was unearthed in Fuhao Tomb of Yin Ruins, Anyang City, Henan Province.

Preserved in Henan Museum

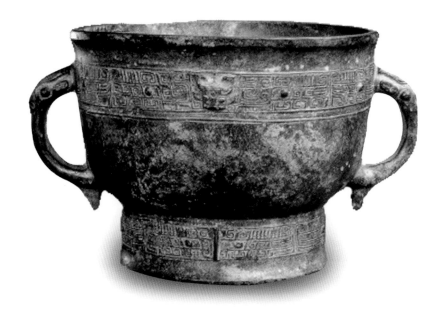

耶簋

商

青铜质

宽 25.5 厘米，高 14.7 厘米

Gui with Character " 耶 "

Shang Dynasty

Bronze

Width 25.5cm/ Height 14.7cm

簋体圆，深腹，双兽耳，方门唇，圈足。颈部正、反两面各有一凸兽首，左、右均饰兽面纹，足饰兽面纹。

故宫博物院藏

This vessel has a round body, a deep belly, two ears with beast designs on them, a square lip, and a ring foot. On the back and front side of the neck, a convex beast head is designed. The left and right parts and the foot of the vessel are decorated with beast face pattern.

Preserved in The Palace Museum

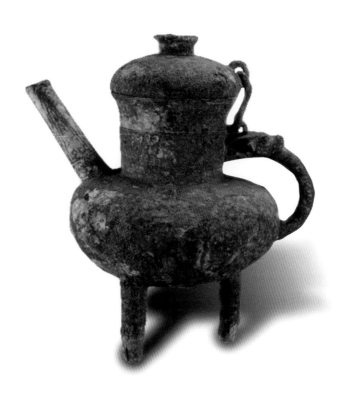

冊冊盉

商

青铜质

宽 30.5 厘米，高 31 厘米

He with Characters "Qu Ce"

Shang Dynasty

Bronze

Width 30.5 cm/ Height 31 cm

腹扁圆，直颈，侈口，有盖。腹有管状流，腹侧有兽首鋬，兽首有链勺盖相连，盖顶有圆握。盖、颈、腹均饰夔纹，流饰叶纹。

故宫博物院藏

The belly of the vessel is in flattened circular shape. There is a straight neck, a flare mouth, and a cover. On the belly, there is a tubular spout and a single ear on one side of the belly in the shape of the head of a sacred animal. The handle is connected with a spoon chain to the cover. There is a round knob on the cover. There is Kui dragon design on the cover, the neck, and the belly. The tubular spout is decorated with leaf-like pattern.

Preserved in The Palace Museum

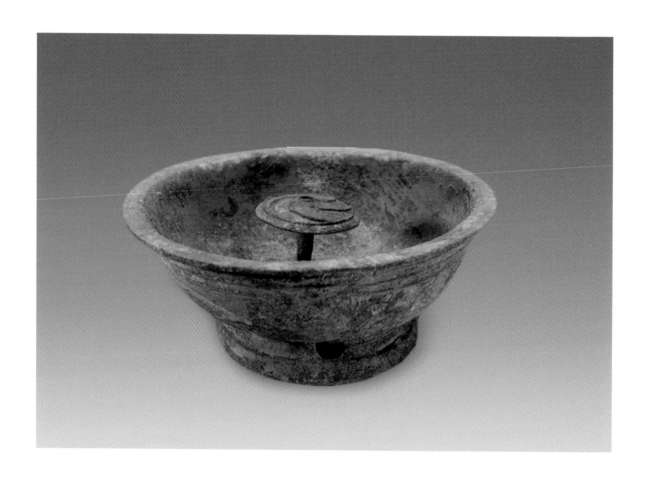

涡纹中柱盂

商

青铜质

口径 29.5 厘米，通高 12 厘米

Yu with Vortex Design and a Central Column

Shang Dynasty

Bronze

Mouth Diameter 29.5 cm/ Height 12 cm

折沿，收腹，圜底，圈足。盂底中央立一菌状柱，柱顶饰涡纹。腹外饰弦纹，圈足上有三个方形镂孔。1982 年河南省郑州向阳回族食品厂商代窑出土。

河南博物院藏

The edges of this ware are folded with downward convergent belly, a round bottom, and a ring foot. There is a mushroom-shaped erect column in the center of the bottom, the top of which is decorated with vortex pattern. The outside of the belly is decorated with bowstring pattern. There are three sculptured square holes on the ring foot. In 1982, it was unearthed in a Kiln of Shang Dynasty in Xiangyang Hui Food Factory in Zhengzhou, Henan Province.

Preserved in Henan Museum

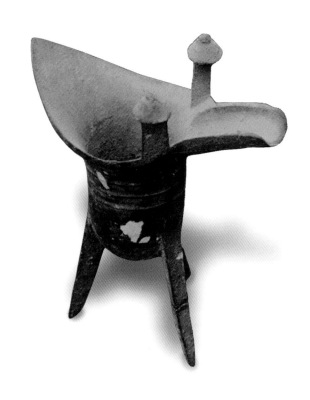

青铜觚（酒杯）

商

青铜质

上口长 15 厘米，上口宽 7.2 厘米，通高 17 厘米，重 0.56 千克

Bronze Gu (Drinking Cup)

Shang Dynasty

Bronze

Length of Upper Mouth 15cm/ Width of Upper Mouth 7.2 cm/ Height 17cm/ Weight 0.56 kg

长身，侈口，口部呈喇叭形。酒器盛行于商代和西周时期。

广东中医药博物馆藏

The vessel has a long body, with a large mouth, like a trumpet's tip. The use of this vessel was popular in the Shang and Western Zhou Dynasties. It served as wine drinking vessel.

Preserved in Guangdong Chinese Medicine Museum

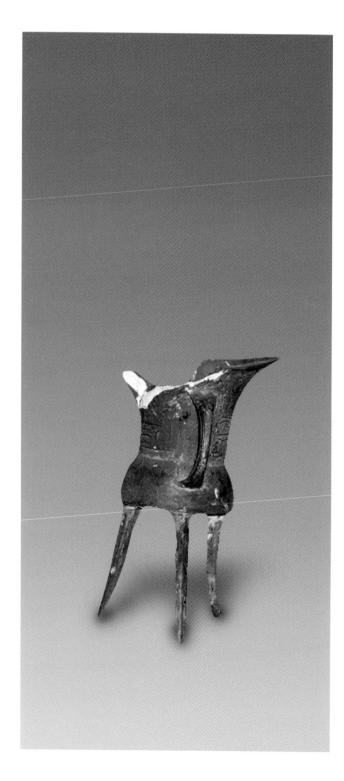

铜爵

商

铜质

口径 14 厘米，底径 7 厘米，通高 17 厘米，

重 2.5 千克

Copper Jue

Shang Dynasty

Copper

Mouth Diameter 14 cm/ Bottom Diameter 7 cm/

Height 17 cm/ Weight 2.5 kg

船形口，直腹，腹上有饕餮纹，带一把，三鼎足。酒器。完整无损。

陕西医史博物馆藏

The vessel has a cymbiform mouth, an erect belly on which there is a Tao Tie pattern (a mythical creature in ancient China), a handle, and tripodal feet. It is a well-preserved wine drinking vessel.

Preserved in Shaanxi Museum of Medical History

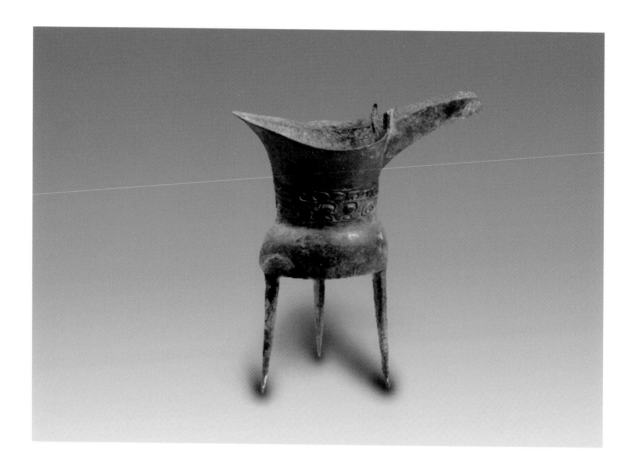

铜爵

商

铜质

高 17 厘米

Copper Jue

Shang Dynasty

Copper

Height 17 cm

束腰，鼓腹，平底，三足细长略向外侈，腹饰饕餮纹。流狭长，尖尾，椭圆形口，流折处两小柱。

南京博物院藏

The vessel has a wasp waist, a drum-shaped belly, and a flat bottom. The tripodal feet are long and slightly stretch outward. The belly is decorated with Tao Tie pattern (a mythical creature in ancient China). The vessel has a long and narrow spout, a sharp tail, and an oval mouth. There are two short pillars in the middle of the mouth of the spout.

Preserved in Nanjing Museum

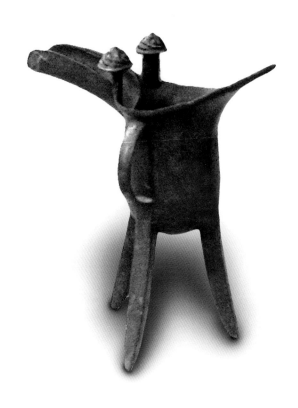

铜爵

商

铜质

口径 18 厘米，通高 20.4 厘米

Copper Jue

Shang Dynasty

Copper

Calibre 18 cm/ Height 20.4 cm

爵形，三足，两柱，带流，桥形耳。爵身有弦纹，耳下阴刻"父乙"两字。饮酒器。造型美观，表面粗糙。保存基本完好。1960 年入藏。

中华医学会 / 上海中医药大学医史博物馆藏

This wine vessel has tripodal feet, two pillars with a spout, and a bridge-shaped ear. There is bowstring pattern on the whole body, and two characters "Fu" and "Yi" are inscribed in intaglio under the ear. This wine drinking vessel is a beautiful in shape but has rough appearances. It is basically in good condition. It was collected in 1960.

Preserved in Chinese Medical Association/ Museum of Chinese Medicine, Shanghai University of Traditional Chinese Medicine

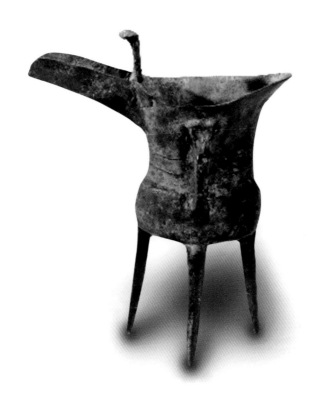

单柱铜爵

商

铜质

通高 17 厘米

Copper Jue with a Single Pillar

Shang Dynasty

Copper

Height 17 cm

前有流，后有尾，流口折处有一菌形单柱。

束腰，上饰两周凸弦纹，下腹鼓出，平底，

三棱锥状足，弧形錾。酒器。此为商代早期

的铜器，在河北地区非常罕见。

河北博物院藏

There is a spout in the front of the body and a tail behind the body. In the break of the spout, there is a single fungus-shaped pillar. The vessel has a wasp waist on which there are two circles of bulgy bowstring patterns. The lower part of the belly swells outward. The vessel also has a flat bottom, a pyramidal three-prism-shaped foot, and an arc-shaped handle. This ware served as a wine-drinking copper vessel in the early Shang Dynasty, and it was very rare in Hebei Province.

Preserved in Hebei Museum

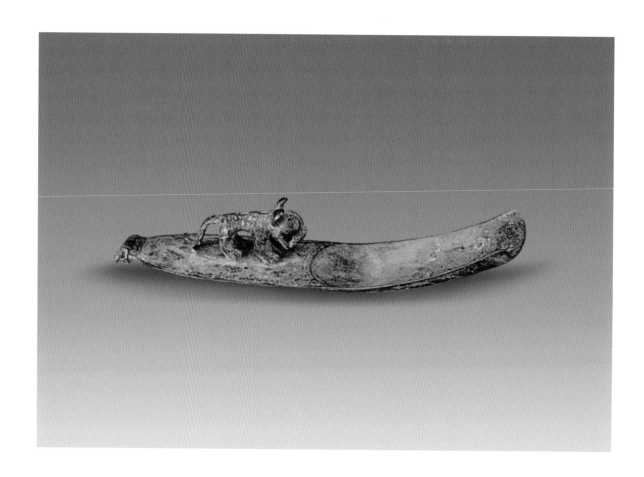

虎饰匕形器

商

青铜质

长 18 厘米，宽 4.5 厘米

Bi with Tiger Design

Shang Dynasty

Bronze

Length 18 cm/ Width 4.5 cm

匕前段上翘呈长方槽状；后段平直厚重，上面置一虎饰，虎呈大头，长尾，口衔物前行状。匕后端渐收细，手柄缺。虎目嵌绿松石，一眼石缺。挹取食器。1959年山西省石楼县桃花村出土。

山西博物院藏

The front part of the vessel tilts upward in the shape of rectangle socket, while the back part is straight and heavy. The back part is decorated with a tiger with a big head and a long tail. The tiger is in the position of walking forward with something in its mouth. The back part of the vessel gradually becomes narrow and there are no handles. One eye of the tiger is embedded with turquoise while the other is short of turquoise. The vessel was used for ladling out food. It was excavated in Taohua Village located in Shilou County, Shanxi, in 1957.

Preserved in Shanxi Museum

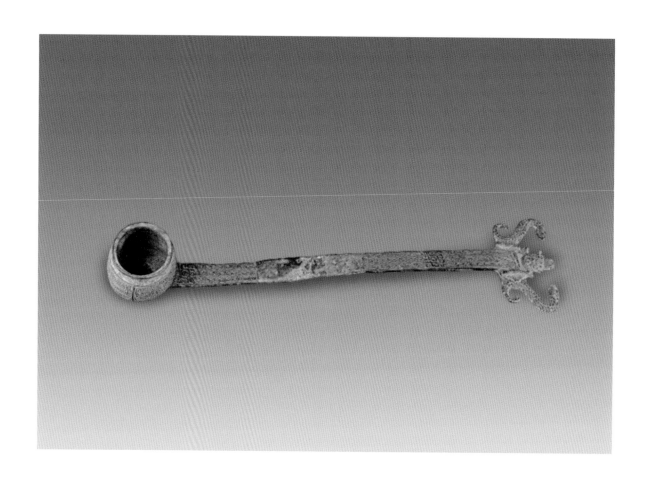

蛇首扁柄斗

商

青铜质

通长 27 厘米，首宽 4.8 厘米

Dou with a Flat Handle with Snake Heads

Shang Dynasty

Bronze

Length 27 cm/ Head Width 4.8 cm

斗呈敛口，鼓腹，平底，罐形。底一侧伸出
扁平长柄，柄首镂雕二蛇戏蛙。斗腹饰云雷
纹地饕餮纹，柄饰云雷纹地夔纹。挹注器。
1957 年山西省石楼县后兰家沟出土。

山西博物院藏

The vessel is in the shape of a jar with convergent
mouth, a swelling belly, and a flat bottom. On one
side of the bottom of the vessel there extends out a
long flat handle. The head of the handle is hollow
engraved with two snakes playing with a frog.
The belly of the vessel is decorated with cloud
and thunder patterns with Tao Tie (a mythical
ferocious animal) pattern as the ground-tint.
The handle is decorated with cloud and thunder
patterns with Kui dragon pattern as the ground-
tint. This vessel was used for bailing. It was
excavated in Houlanjiagou, Shilou County,
Shanxi in 1957.

Preserved in Shanxi Museum

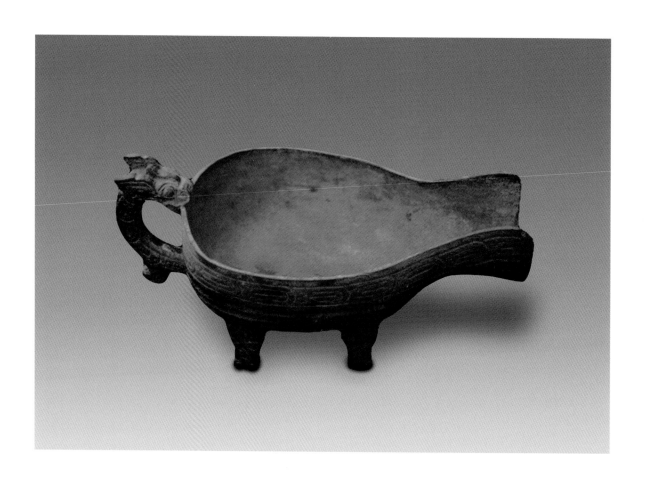

青铜匜

商

青铜质

流至出水口长 23 厘米，宽 13 厘米，出水口宽 5.8 厘米，通高 15.1 厘米，腹深 6.8 厘米

Bronze Yi

Shang Dynasty

Bronze

Length 23 cm /Width 5.8 cm/ Spout Width 5.8 cm/ Height 15.1 cm/ Depth 6.8 cm

洗器，是中国古代水器，与盘配套使用，为古代卫生保健用品。有铭文铸于内底 2 行 12 个字。

广东中医药博物馆藏

The bronze artifact was used as a washer in ancient China. Together with plates when used, it belonged to the health care products in the past. In the inner bottom of the bronze artifact, there is an inscription of 12 characters in 2 lines.

Preserved in Guangdong Chinese Medicine Museum

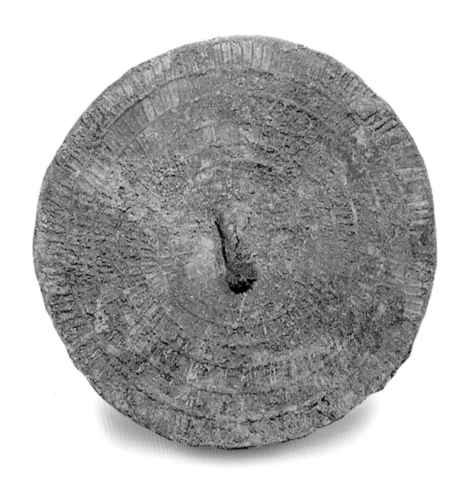

铜镜

商

铜质

直径 12.5 厘米，厚 0.4 厘米

背面周缘饰两圈凸弦纹，内有一圈排列整齐的小乳钉纹，中心部位饰以叶脉纹，靠钮外又有一圈凸弦纹。生活用具。1976 年河南安阳殷墟妇好墓出土。

殷墟博物馆藏

Bronze Mirror

Shang Dynasty

Copper

Diameter 12.5 cm/ Thickness 0.4 cm

The edge at the rear of the mirror is decorated with raised bowstring patterns in two concentric circles. Within these, small papillae are lined up in a smaller circle. The center of this mirror is decorated with leaf veins pattern surrounded by another circle of convex bowstring patterns. It was commonly utilized in daily life in ancient times. It was excavated in the Tomb of Fuhao, Anyang City, Henan Province, in 1976.

Preserved in Yinxu Museum

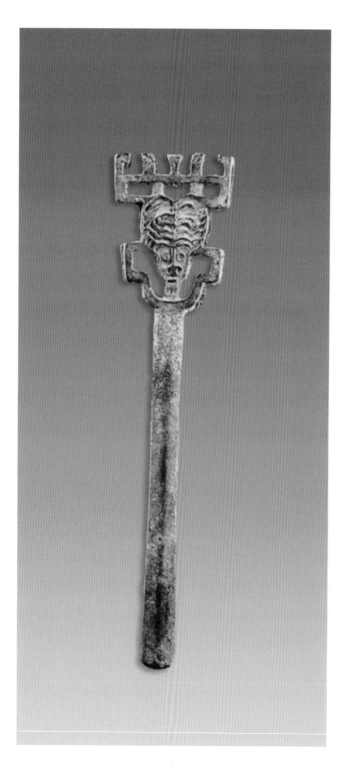

人首笄形器

商

青铜质

长 16.5 厘米，首宽 4 厘米

Ancient Hair Clasp

Shang Dynasty

Bronze

Length 16.5 cm/ Head Width 4 cm

笄为扁长条形，略弧。一端为扁平笄首，正
面呈人像，两侧镂空边框。高盘发双分，上
饰波状纹，顶呈齿状高冠。束发器。1959 年
山西省忻县连寺沟牛子坪出土。

山西博物院藏

The clasp is flat and long with a bit of an arc.
On one end of the clasp there is a flat head
engraved to resemble a woman's face. The hair
is symmetrically divided into two parts, highly
coiled and in the design of wave-like patterns.
The top of the clasp is in the shape of teeth and a
high crest and the frame of the clasp is hollowed
out. It was utilized as a hair tie. It was excavated
in Niuziping, Liansi of Qixian County, Shanxi
Province.

Preserved in Shanxi Museum

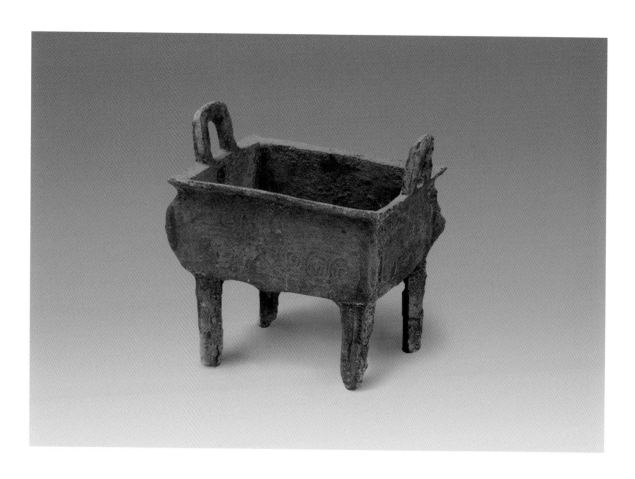

青铜方鼎

西周早期

青铜质

通高 18 厘米

Bronze Quadripod Caldron

Early Western Zhou Dynasty

Bronze

Height 18 cm

直耳，方沿，柱足。鼎腹长方形，饰两周云纹带，两端为雷纹，四角有扉棱。云雷纹在中原铜器上常作地纹以烘托主纹，在吴国青铜器上则常用做主纹，颇具朴素平淡之风格。器外底四周亦残留有铸造痕迹。溧水乌山岗沿山出土。

镇江博物馆藏

The quadripod has prick ears, square edges, columnar legs and a rectangular belly surrounded by two bands of whorled pattern with squared whorled decorations on both ends. There are leaf ridges on the four corners of the vessel. On the bronze vessels in central plains region of China, cloud and thunder pattern is often used as ground-tint to make the main pattern stand out. However, on the bronzes of the state of Wu, it is often used as the main pattern, and it displays a style of simplicity. Around the outer bottom, there still remain the traces of casting. It was unearthed from Gangyan Mountain, Wushan Town, Lishui District.

Preserved in Zhenjiang Museum

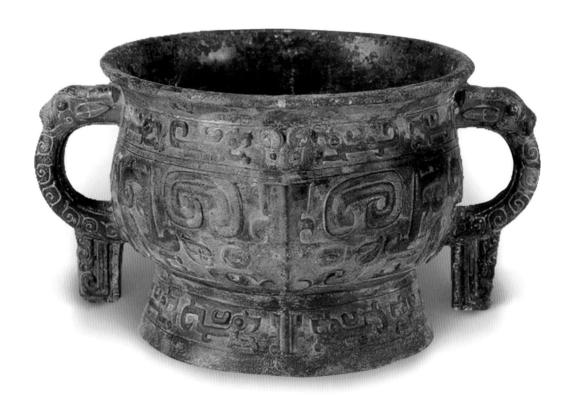

兽面纹五耳鼎

西周早期

青铜质

口径 83 厘米，高 122 厘米，重 226 千克

鼎是商周青铜礼器中的重要的食器，有烹煮
肉食、实牲祭祀和宴飨等各种用途。

陕西历史博物馆藏

Five Ears Ding with Animal Mask Pattern

Early Western Zhou Dynasty

Bronze

Mouth Diameter 83 cm/ Height 122 cm/ Weight 226 kg

Ding is an important cooking vessel among bronze ritual vessels in the Shang and Zhou Dynasties. It served to cook meat or food or to be used in sacrifice rituals or banquets.

Preserved in Shaanxi History Museum

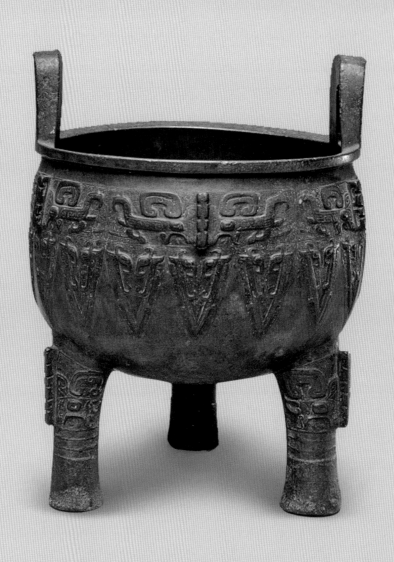

兽面纹鼎

西周早期

青铜质

宽 33.7 厘米，通高 41.4 厘米，重 18.52 千克

立耳，平沿外折，柱足。纹饰分三组，口下呈兽面纹，腹部施垂叶云纹，足根饰兽面，相互照应，显得十分得体。此鼎造型凝重，工艺精湛，是西周早期的一件艺术珍品。清宫旧藏。

故宫博物院藏

Tripod with Animal Mask Pattern

Early Western Zhou Dynasty

Bronze

Width 33.7 cm/ Height 41.4 cm/ Weight 18.52 kg

The tripod has prick ears, folded edges, and columnar legs. There are three groups of decorations on the tripod. Below the rim of the mouth on the outside there are animal-mask designs; on the belly there is hanging leaf and cloud pattern, and the heels are decorated with animal-mask designs. The three groups of pattern are in harmony with each other. With its dignified design and exquisite workmanship, this tripod is a treasure of art from the early Western Zhou Dynasty. It is an antique in the heritage of the imperial palace of the Qing Dynasty.

Preserved in The Palace Museum

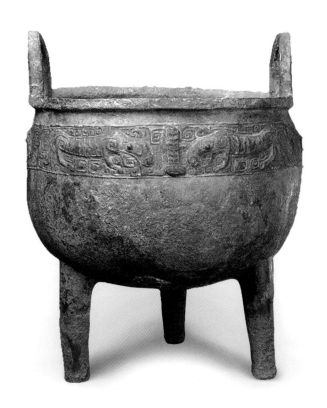

虎纹鼎

西周早期

青铜质

宽 33 厘米，通高 40.9 厘米，重 9.68 千克

Tripod with Tiger Pattern

Early Western Zhou Dynasty

Bronze

Width 33 cm/ Height 40.9 cm/ Weight 9.68 kg

器壁较薄，立耳，口沿外折，中腹微鼓，柱足较细。口下花纹深镂细刻，层次分明。主体虎纹突出器表，近于浮雕，其上又勾勒阳线花纹。地纹用纤细的云雷纹，有机地和主体花纹相配合。1957 年 3 月收购。

故宫博物院藏

The tripod has a thin wall, two prick ears, and outward folded edges, a slightly bulged belly and three thin columnar legs. Below the rim of the mouth on the outside, there is decorative pattern deeply and elaborately engraved and well arranged. The pattern of tiger rises up from the body surface like relief, and on it there are designs of flowers outlined with raised lines. The background designs are fine cloud and thunder patterns, and they match the main flower designs perfectly. The tripod was acquired in March 1957.

Preserved in The Palace Museum

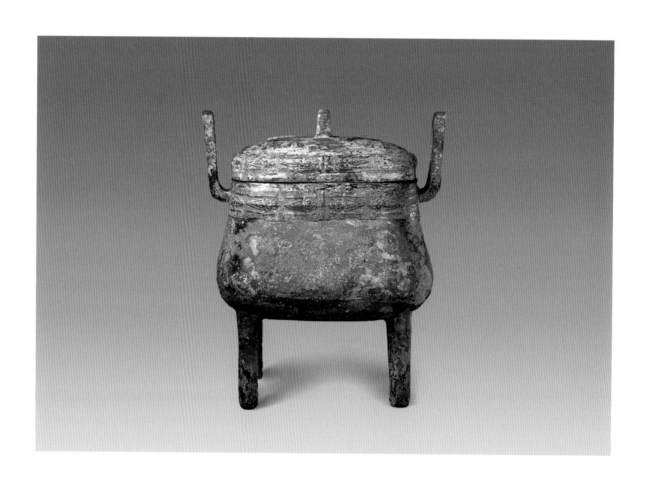

作宝彝方鼎

西周早期

青铜质

宽 24.4 厘米，通高 27.1 厘米，重 3.3 千克

Quadripod Caldron with Characters "Zuo Bao Yi"

Early Western Zhou Dynasty

Bronze

Width 24.4 cm/ Height 27.1 cm/ Weight 3.3 kg

造型规整新颖，独具风格。附耳，柱足，直
口有盖，下腹倾垂。鼎盖中鼻钮，盖沿和器
颈部饰云雷纹衬地的带状蝉纹。内底和盖内
铸相同的铭文 3 字"作宝彝"。清宫旧藏。

故宫博物院藏

The modeling of the tripod is clear, neat and
novel with a unique style. It has two accessory
ears, three columnar legs, a straight mouth
with a cover, and a deflexed belly. In the center
of the cover, there is a nasal knob. The edge
of the cover and the neck of the quadripod
are decorated with banded cicada designs
with cloud and thunder pattern as supporting
base. There is an inscription of the same three
characters "Zuo Bao Yi" on the bottom inside
the tripod and on the inner side of the cover.
The quadripod belongs to the collection of the
imperial palace of the Qing Dynasty.

Preserved in The Palace Museum

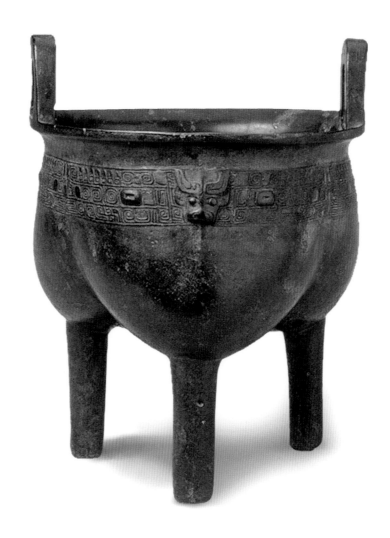

史斿父鼎

西周早期

青铜质

宽 19.5 厘米，通高 25 厘米，重 2.52 千克

Tripod with Characters "Shi You Fu"

Early Western Zhou Dynasty

Bronze

Width 19.5 cm/ Height 25 cm/ Weight 2.52 kg

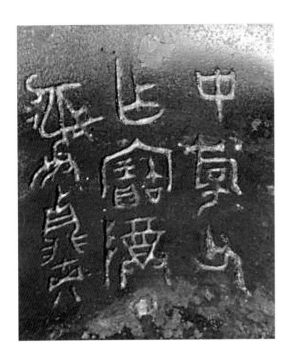
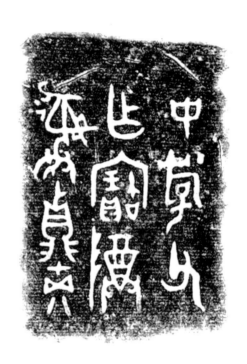

分裆，实足，立耳，口微侈。颈部饰列旗兽面纹，兽面中部附饰浮雕牺首。内壁铸铭文 3 行 9 字，记史
斿父做鼎。铭后所附数字是八卦符号，表明铸造此鼎时曾经进行一次卜筮。1957 年收购。

故宫博物院藏

The tripod has an open crotch, three solid legs, prick ears, and a mouth that slightly extends outward. Its crotch is similar to that of the cooking vessel. The neck is decorated with animal-mask designs with feather-shaped pattern on the top of their forehead; and in the center of the animal-mask, there is a decoration of an animal head in relief for sacrifice. On the inner wall of the tripod, there are 9 characters in 3 lines recording that Shi You Fu made this tripod. The numbers attached to the inscription stand for symbols of the Eight Diagrams, indicating that there was a divination when this tripod was to be made. The tripod was acquired in 1957.

Preserved in The Palace Museum

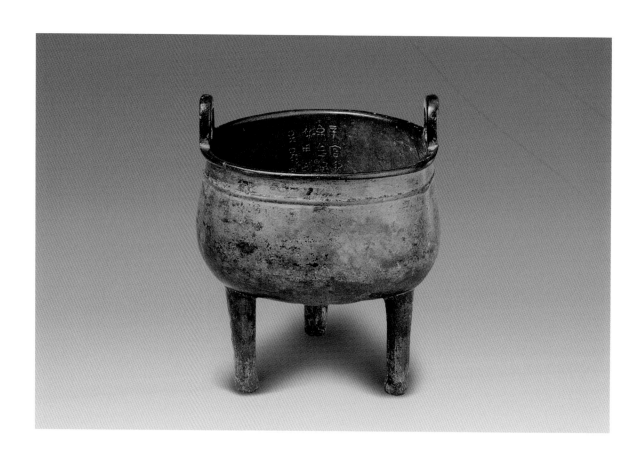

舍父鼎

西周早期

青铜质

宽 14.8 厘米，通高 17 厘米，重 0.8 千克

Tripod with Characters "She Fu"

Early Western Zhou Dynasty

Bronze

Width 14.8 cm/ Height 17 cm/ Weight 0.8 kg

立耳，垂腹，底近平，柱足。口沿下有弦纹
一道。内壁一侧铸铭文 22 字，记辛宫赏赐
给舍父帛和铜块，为宣扬辛宫的美意做了这
件宝鼎，子孙后代永远宝用它。1957 年收购。

故宫博物院藏

The tripod has two prick ears, a pot-shaped
belly, a bottom that is almost flat, and three
columnar legs. Below the rim of the mouth
on the outside, there is a streak of raised line
design. On one side of the inner wall, there is
an inscription of 22 characters that record why
this tripod was cast: Xin Gong bestowed silk
and copper masses to She Fu as reward. To
publicize the kindness of Xin Gong, this tripod
was cast so that his descendants would be able to
use it forever. The tripod was acquired in 1957.
Preserved in The Palace Museum

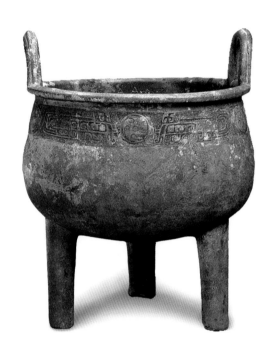

伯和鼎

西周早期

青铜质

宽 25 厘米，通高 30 厘米，重 5.74 千克

Tripod with Characters "Bo He"

Early Western Zhou Dynasty

Bronze

Width 25 cm/ Height 30 cm/ Weight 5.74 kg

绚状立耳，方唇外折，鼓腹，柱足。口沿下
有四个圆涡纹，其间分布两两相对的三组以
分尾夔纹组成的兽面纹。内壁一侧铸铭文 3
行 10 字，记伯和为其召伯父辛做鼎。1959
年收购。

故宫博物院藏

The tripod has two rope-shaped prick ears,
a square lip that is folded outward, a bulged
belly, and three columnar legs. Below the rim
of the mouth on the outside, there are four
circular vortex patterns between which there
are three groups of face-to-face animal-mask
designs with separate tails decorated with
designs of "Kui", a monster in fable. On one
side of the inner wall, there is an inscription of
10 characters in 3 lines that record that Bo He
made the tripod for Zhao Bo Fu Xin. The tripod
was acquired in 1959.

Preserved in The Palace Museum

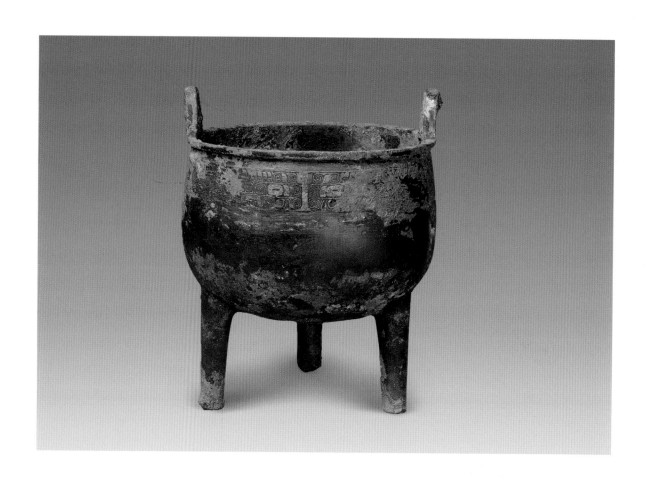

寓鼎

西周早期

青铜质

宽 22.2 厘米，通高 26.5 厘米，重 3.76 千克

Tripod with Character "Yu"

Early Western Zhou Dynasty

Bronze

Width 22.2 cm/ Height 26.5 cm/ Weight 3.76 kg

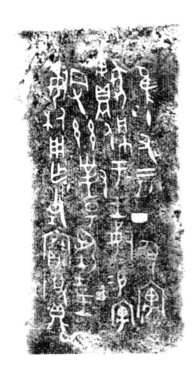

深圆腹，三柱足，二直耳。口沿下饰兽面纹带，纹带的上列出现了一排旗状图案。鼎内壁有铭文4行，共30字。1956年国家文物局调拨。

故宫博物院藏

The tripod has a deep round belly, three columnar legs, and two prick ears. Below the rim of the mouth on the outside, there is a band of animal mask designs. Above the decoration band, there is a row of flag-shaped pattern. In the inner wall of the tripod, there is a 30-character inscription in 4 lines. The tripod was allocated from State Administration of Cultural Heritage in 1956.

Preserved in The Palace Museum

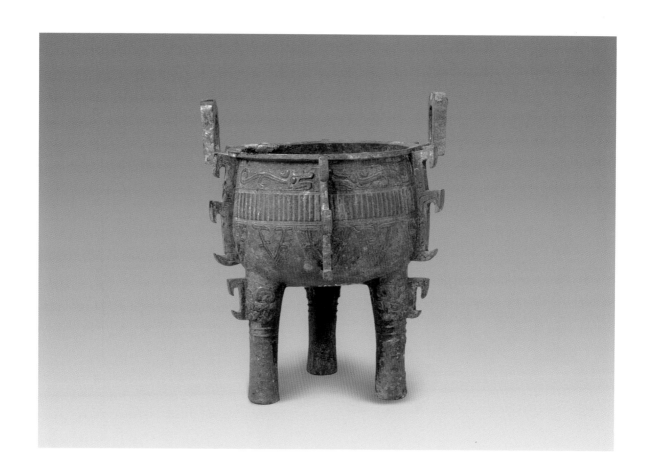

田田 鼎

西周早期

青铜质

宽 20 厘米，通高 23 厘米，重 2.76 千克

Tripod with Character "田田"

Early Western Zhou Dynasty

Bronze

Width 20 cm/ Height 23 cm/ Weight 2.76 kg

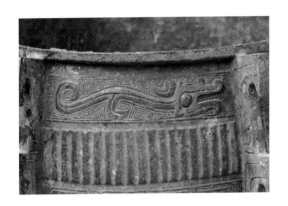

圆腹，二直耳，三足形状近似马蹄形，器体棱脊四起。全身满施花纹，深镂细刻，富丽堂皇。颈部饰云雷纹填地的对夔纹，夔形张口卷尾，腹下部是三角形的垂叶纹，腹中部则采用简洁的直线纹作装饰。足的根部饰以兽面。鼎内铸一"𤰔"字。传陕西宝鸡出土，1957 年李德全先生捐献。

故宫博物院藏

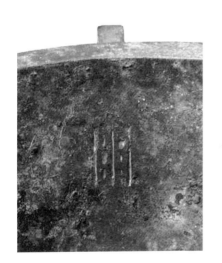

The tripod has a round belly, two prick ears, three legs shaped like a horseshoe, and four ridges on the body. All over the tripod, there are flower designs, deeply and finely engraved, displaying a sense of magnificence. There is symmetrical design of Kui, a one-legged monster in fable, on the neck, with cloud and thunder pattern as the supporting base. The Kui opens its mouth and curls its tail. The central part of the belly is decorated with a simple pattern of lines, and the lower part of the belly is cast with triangular hanging leaf patterns. The end of the legs is decorated with animal-mask design. There is an inscription of the character "𤰔" inside the tripod. It is said that the tripod was unearthed in Baoji, Shaanxi Province. It was donated to the museum by Mr. Li Dequan in 1957. Preserved in The Palace Museum

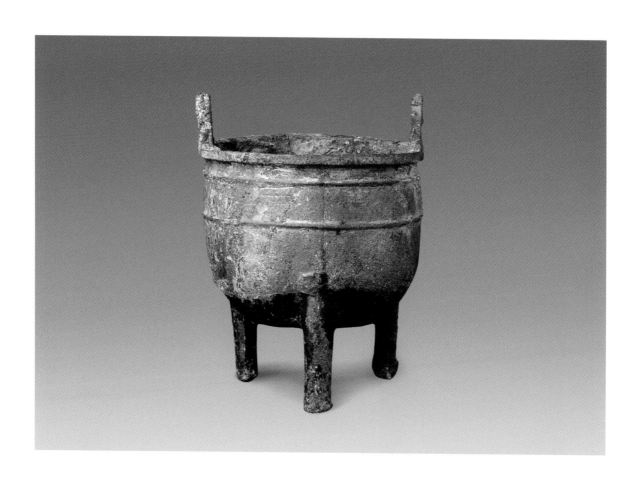

嬴霝德鼎

西周早期

青铜质

宽 8.3 厘米，通高 10.6 厘米，重 0.36 千克

Tripod with Characters "Ying Ling De"

Early Western Zhou Dynasty

Bronze

Width 8.3 cm/ Height 10.6 cm/ Weight 0.36 kg

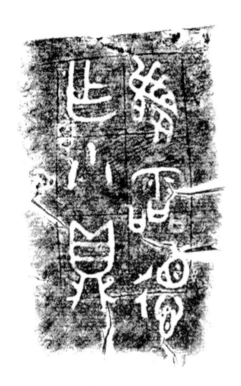

深圆腹，三柱足较短，平沿外折，二直耳，腹饰二道弦纹。鼎内铸有铭文 2 行 6 字，记赢霝德做此小鼎。自铭"小鼎"者，较为少见。1956 年国家文物局调拨。

故宫博物院藏

The tripod has a deep round belly, three short columnar legs, a flat edge that folds outward, two prick ears, and two streaks of string pattern decorated on the belly. Inside the tripod, there is a 6-character inscription in two lines, recording that Ying Ling De made this small tripod. It is rare that the caster inscribed the tripod he made as "small tripod". The tripod was allocated from State Administration of Cultural Heritage in 1956.

Preserved in The Palace Museum

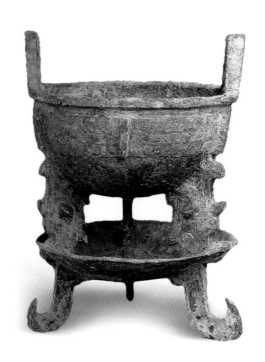

有盘鼎

西周早期

青铜质

宽 16.4 厘米，通高 20.2 厘米，重 2.26 千克

Tripod with a Plate-like Partition

Early Western Zhou Dynasty

Bronze

Width 16.4 cm/ Height 20.2 cm/ Weight 2.26 kg

圆形，浅腹，二直耳，三夔形扁足，足中部
有隔似盘，此盘的用途是置炭火。颈部饰兽
面纹带，兽面中间凸起一道扉棱，好像是兽
面的鼻子。1956 年国家文物局调拨。

故宫博物院藏

The tripod is round in shape with a shallow
belly, two prick ears, and three flat legs shaped
like a Kui, a legendary monster. In the middle
of the legs, there is a plate-like partition, which
serves to hold burning charcoal. The neck is
decorated with a band of animal-mask designs
with a vertical leaf ridge in its middle, like
the nose of the animal mask. The tripod was
allocated from State Administration of Cultural
Heritage in 1956.

Preserved in The Palace Museum

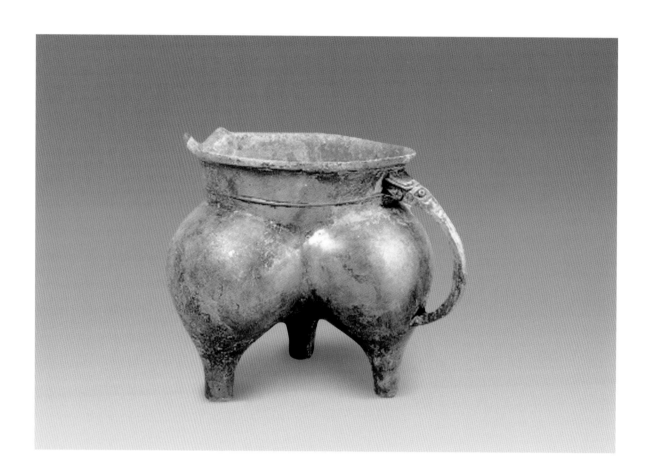

青铜单耳有流鬲

西周早期 (前 1000—前 950)

青铜质

口径 15.4 厘米，高 17 厘米

Bronze Li with a Looped Handle and a Peaked Spout

Early Western Zhou Dynasty (1000 B.C.–950 B.C.)

Bronze

Mouth Diameter 15.4 cm/ Height 17 cm

此鬲带流与鋬，功能较为进步。3条肥硕的
空袋足界限分明，裆部分开，即所谓"分裆鬲"。
器表素雅光洁。山西省曲沃县曲村晋国墓地
出土。

北京大学赛克勒考古与艺术博物馆藏

This vessel is advanced in its functions for it
has a loop handle and a peaked spout. It used
to serve as a cooking vessel with separated
crotch due to its three stout hollow bag-like legs
with clear boundaries and a separated crotch.
The surface is simple, elegant and smooth. The
cooking vessel was unearthed in the cemetery of
Jin State in Qu Village, Quwo County, Shanxi
Province.

Preserved in Arthur M. Sackler Museum of Art
and Archaeology at Peking University

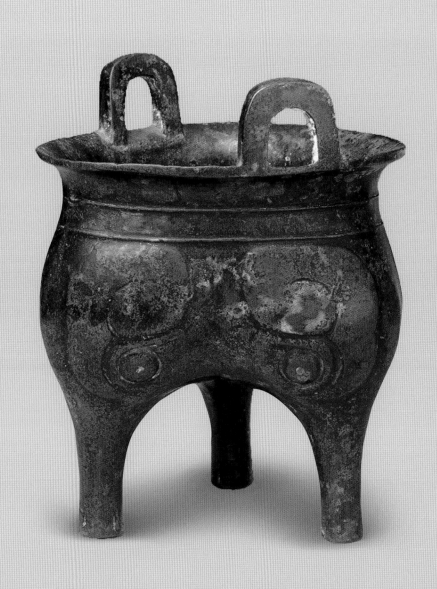

作宝尊彝鬲

西周早期

青铜质

宽 13.5 厘米，通高 16 厘米，重 0.92 千克

立耳分裆式鬲。侈口，圆唇，足饰象首纹，装饰十分简朴。器内有铭文 4 字。1958 年收购。

故宫博物院藏

Li with Characters "Zuo Bao Zun Yi"

Early Western Zhou Dynasty

Bronze

Width 13.5 cm/ Height 16 cm/ Weight 0.92 kg

This cooking vessel has prick ears, a separated crotch, a large mouth and round lips. The design of an elephant head is decorated on its legs, and the decoration is simple and plain. An inscription of 4 words is cast inside the vessel. It was acquired in 1958.

Preserved in The Palace Museum

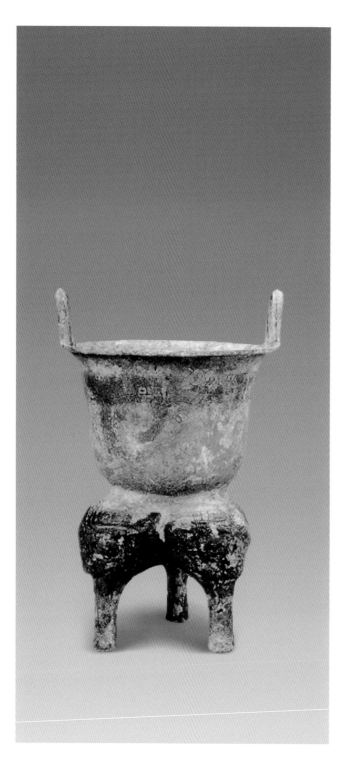

青铜甗

西周早期 (前 1000—前 950)

青铜质

口径 33.8 厘米，高 40.3 厘米

Bronze Yan

Early Western Zhou Dynasty (1000 B.C–950 B.C)

Bronze

Mouth Diameter 33.8 cm/ Height 40.3 cm

西周早期的青铜甗在形态上与商代晚期区别
不大，也是上甑下鬲连铸而成。此件设计扩
大了烧火空间与蒸食的容量。浮雕极富层次
感。山西省曲沃县曲村晋国墓地出土。

北京大学赛克勒考古与艺术博物馆藏

The bronze Yan, a steaming cookers in early
Western Zhou Dynasty, has no great differences
with the steaming cookers of Late Shang
Dynasty which are also connected by a Zeng
steamer caldron (upper part) and Li cooking
vessel (lower part). The designing of this
steaming vessel enlarges the space of burning
fire and the volume of steamed food. The relief
gives people a good sense of layers. It was
unearthed in the tomb of Jin State in Qu Village,
Quwo County, Shanxi Province.
Preserved in Arthur M. Sackler Museum of Art
and Archaeology at Peking University

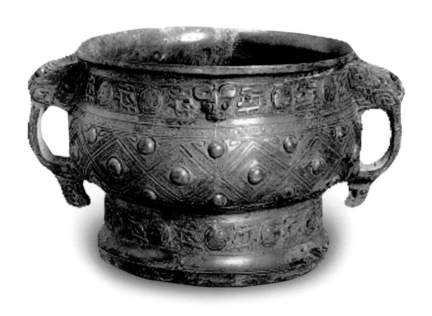

青铜簋

西周早期（前 1000—前 950）

青铜质

口径 18.5 厘米，腹径 19.8 厘米，高 14.1 厘米

Bronze Gui

Early Western Zhou Dynasty (1000 B.C.–950B.C.)

Bronze

Mouth Diameter18.5 cm /Belly Diameter 19.8 cm/ Height 14.1 cm

此件铸造技艺精湛，画面极具动感，为西周早期青铜铸造业的典范之作。内壁底面铸有"乍（作）宝彝"3字铭文。商周时期盛黍稷稻粱的器皿，容量为1~2升。山西省曲沃县曲晋村国墓地出土。

北京大学赛克勒考古与艺术博物馆藏

The vessel displays a superb casting technique with a strong sense of animation for the picture. It is a classic model work of the foundry industry of bronzeware in early Western Zhou Dynasty. The inner wall is cast with an inscription of 3 characters "Zuo Bao Yi". It is a popular container which used to be used for containing wheat, rice, and sorghum, in Shang and Western Zhou Dynasties. The size of volume is about 1–2 L. It was unearthed in the tomb of Jin State in Qu Village, Quwo County, Shanxi Province.

Preserved in Arthur M. Sackler Museum of Art and Archaeology at Peking University

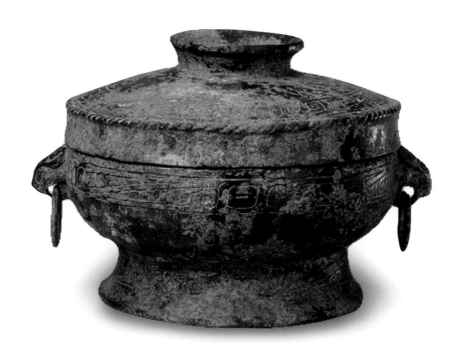

遹遜父癸簋

西周早期

青铜质

宽 26.5 厘米，通高 17 厘米，重 2.73 千克

Gui with Characters Including " 遜 "

Early Western Zhou Dynasty

Bronze

Width 26.5 cm/ Height 17 cm/ Weight 2.73 kg

弇口，圆腹，腹上有一对兽头衔环耳，盖口与器相合，圈足外侈。器腹、盖上与圈足均饰目雷纹。盖和器均有铭文9字。1958年收购。

故宫博物院藏

This vessel has a small mouth and a round belly. There is a pair of beast-shaped handles on the sides of the belly. The mouth of the cover matches with the body. The ring foot is flared. The belly, cover and flared foot of this vessel are all decorated with eye-like pattern intertwined with thunder patterns. On both of the cover and body, there is an inscription of 9 characters. It was acquired in 1958.

Preserved in The Palace Museum

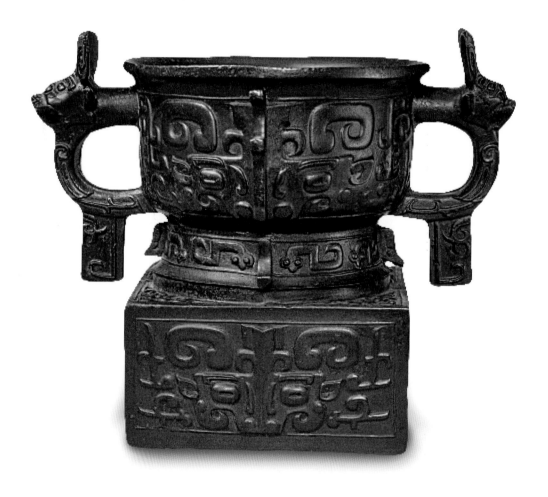

作宝彝簋

西周早期

青铜质

宽 30.7 厘米，通高 25.5 厘米，重 5.42 千克

侈口，方唇，鼓腹，圈足下有座。双耳做成兽首屈舌形，垂珥较长，兽耳高出器口。腹部和方座均饰大兽面，近似浮雕，凸目张口，神态威严，腹上兽面中部尚突起扉棱。圈足饰两两相对的蚕纹，中隔扉棱。造型庄重，装饰富丽，是西周早期流行的方座簋。内底铸"作宝彝"3 字，无做器人名。清宫旧物（原藏颐和园）。

故宫博物院藏

Gui with Characters "Zuo Bao Yi"

Early Western Zhou Dynasty

Bronze

Width 30.7 cm/ Height 25.5 cm/ Weight 5.42 kg

The vessel has a flared mouth with a squared lip and a swelling belly. There is a squared pedestal under the ring foot. The two handles are cast into a shape of beast head with curled tongue. The decorations of the handles are long. The beast-shaped handles stand higher than the level of the mouth. The belly and square pedestal are decorated with large beast face pattern, similar to relief. The beast has bulged eyes, an opened mouth with a dignified expression. On the center of the beast face of the belly, there is a protuberant ridge. The ring foot is decorated with symmetrical patterns of silkworm that alternate with ridges. This design of the vessel is solemn with magnificent ornamentation. This Gui with its square pedestal was popular in early Western Zhou Dynasty. The inner side of the bottom is cast with an inscription of 3 characters "Zuo Bao Yi", but without casting the name of the craftsman. This used to be a vessel of the imperial palace of the Qing Dynasty and was originally preserved in the Summer Palace.

Preserved in The Palace Museum

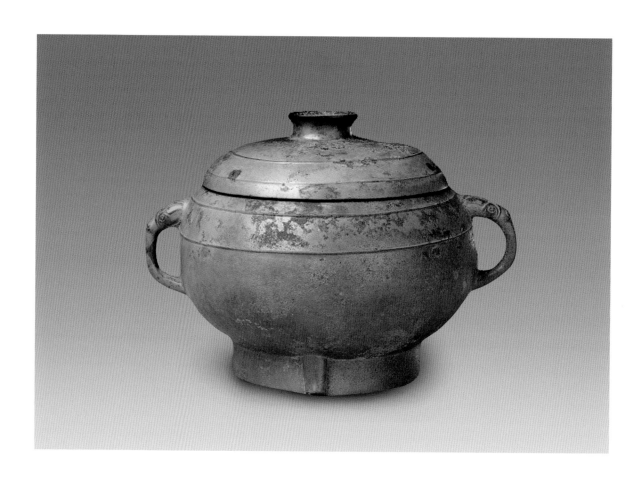

覗父壬簋

西周早期

青铜质

宽 24.7 厘米，通高 16.1 厘米，重 1.76 千克

Gui with Characters Including "覗"

Early Western Zhou Dynasty

Bronze

Width 24.7 cm/ Height 16.1 cm/ Weight 1.76 kg

盖与器子母合口，盖上有喇叭形捉手。腹两侧铸兽耳，圈足。盖沿及器口沿各施弦纹两道。盖内与器底对铭，各铸 8 字，记觥为父壬做器，铭末"射"字为其族名。1958 年 3 月 6 日收购。

　　　　　　　　　故宫博物院藏

The cover is fit with the mouth of the vessel, and there is a trumpet-shaped knob on the cover. On both sides of the belly, there is an ear shaped like a beast. The vessel has a ring foot. The edge of the cover and the edge of the mouth both have two circles of string patterns. The 8-character inscription of inner side of the cover corresponds with 8-character inscription of inner side of the bottom of the vessel, recording that the person who made this precious vessel in memory of Father Ren. The character "She" at the end of the inscription is the name of his clan. The vessel was collected on March 6, 1958.

Preserved in The Palace Museum

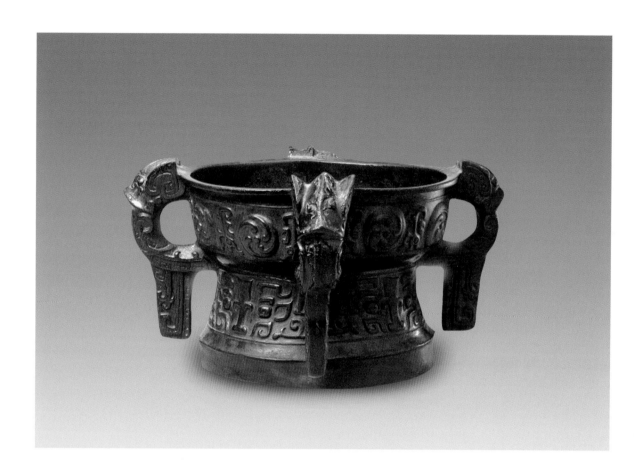

荣簋

西周早期

青铜质

宽 28.8 厘米，通高 14.8 厘米，重 1 千克

Gui with Character "Rong"

Early Western Zhou Dynasty

Bronze

Width 28.8 cm/ Height 14.8 cm/ Weight 1 kg

圆浅腹，平沿，高圈足。四兽耳，每耳的兽头均高出口沿，并有下垂的长方形小珥，小珥近地，上面雕饰兽尾、兽足，使耳与小珥在构图上成为一个整体。腹部饰圆涡纹和夔纹，夔呈倒置状，圈足饰有四组兽面纹。簋内底有铭文 5 行 30 字。清宫旧藏。

故宫博物院藏

The vessel has a round and shallow belly, a flat edge, a high ring foot and four beast-shaped handles. Each beast head on the handle stands higher than the level of the mouth and has small rectangular dropping decorations. The dropping decoration almost reaches the ground, on which beast tail and beast feet are designed so that the handles are integrated with the small dropping decoration as a whole in structure. The belly is decorated with vortex patterns and inverted Kui dragon patterns. The ring foot is decorated with four groups of beast face patterns. There is an inscription of 30 characters in 5 lines on the inner bottom of this vessel. It was a vessel of the imperial palace of the Qing Dynasty. Preserved in The Palace Museum

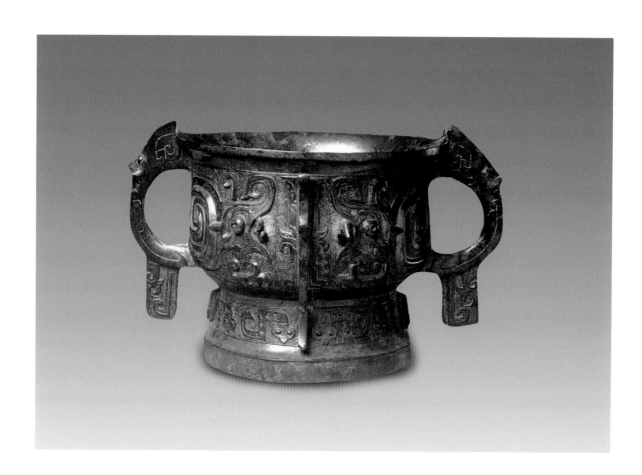

团龙纹簋

西周早期

青铜质

宽 27.3 厘米，通高 15.8 厘米，重 2.24 千克

Gui with Curled-up Dragons Designs

Early Western Zhou Dynasty

Bronze

Width 27.8 cm/ Height 15.8 cm/ Weight 2.2 kg

圆腹，侈口，圈足。腹有二兽耳垂珥。腹饰浮雕状团龙纹，两两对峙，鼻上卷，张口，双齿外露，身尾卷曲。圈足施弓身卷尾蚕纹。通体用细云雷纹为地。清宫旧藏。

故宫博物院藏

The vessel has a round belly, a flared big mouth, and a ring foot. The belly has two beast handles with a dropping decoration, and is decorated with curled-up dragons patterns in relief with two dragons opposing each other, noses curling upward, mouth opening, teeth exposed to the outside, the body and the tail curling. The ring foot is decorated with patterns of silkworm that bends low its body and curls its tail. The whole body is filled with thin cloud and thunder pattern. The vessel used to be an item of the imperial palace of the Qing Dynasty.

Preserved in The Palace Museum

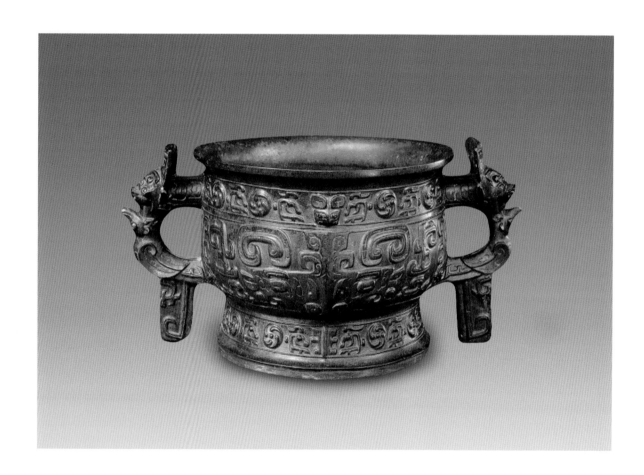

堇临簋

西周早期

青铜质

宽 33.5 厘米，通高 16.7 厘米，重 3.66 千克

Gui with Characters "Jin Lin"

Early Western Zhou Dynasty

Bronze

Width 33.5 cm/ Height 16.7 cm/ Weight 3.66 kg

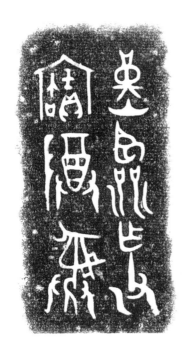

双耳簋，在隆起的腹部上用大兽面纹来做装饰。颈部和圈足也都有一道纹带，用变体夔纹和涡纹相间，颈部中间还加饰浮雕牺首。此簋的耳部装饰十分突出，圆形的耳上部雕铸兽头，双角耸立，突出的上唇下露出 2 颗锐利的长牙。耳的大部又雕刻出一个鸟。鸟头抵在牺首的颜下，突出的鸟嘴向下弯曲，鸟身和两翼略作弧形，鸟尾与器相合，在耳下方的长方形垂珥上，则刻出鸟足和羽毛。簋内底有铭文 8 字，记堇临做此簋的目的是祭祀父乙。清宫旧藏。

故宫博物院藏

This vessel has two handles. The swelling belly is decorated with large beast face patterns. There is a band of whorl designs that alternate with transformed Kui dragon designs and vortex patterns on both the neck and the ring foot, and there are embossed patterns of cattle head on the middle of neck. The upper part of the two round handles is decorated with a beast head with its two horns erecting, and two sharp teeth exposed from the protruding upper lip. The most part of the handle is decorated with a bird, with its head lying against the submaxillary region of the beast head. The protruding bird beak bends downward, the bird body and the wings are designed in the shape of an arch. Its tail meets with the vessel. On the rectangular dropping decoration of the lower part of the handle, there is sculpture of bird feet and features. The 8 characters cast on the inside bottom of the vessel record that Jin Lin made this precious vessel in memory of Father Yi. The vessel used to be an antique of the imperial palace of the Qing Dynasty and was originally preserved in the Summer Palace.

Preserved in The Palace Museum

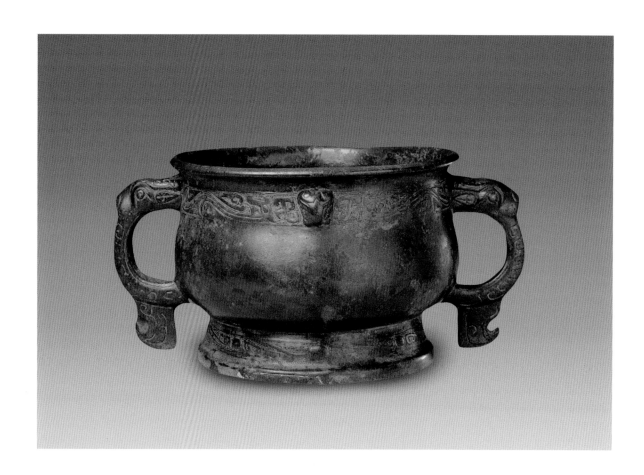

易旁簋

西周早期

青铜质

宽 29.2 厘米，通高 14.3 厘米，重 2.7 千克

Gui Characters including " 易 "

Early Western Zhou Dynasty

Bronze

Width 29.2 cm/ Height 14.3 cm/ Weight 2.7 kg

侈口，圆腹，高圈足，兽首耳下有垂珥。口下饰垂冠回首夔龙。中间用两个浮雕牺首相隔。圈足饰长体夔龙，均用云雷纹填地。内底铭文 3 行 24 字。1959 年入藏。

故宫博物院藏

The container has a wide flared mouth and a round belly with a high ring foot. There is a dropping decoration under each handle of the bronze vessel shaped in an animal head. Below the rim of the mouth, a head-turning Kui dragon with dropping crest is decorated. Two heads of sacrificial beasts in relief oppose each other on the opposite side of the Kui dragon pattern. The ring foot is decorated with a long-body Kui dragon and filled with cloud and thunder patterns as the ground design. The inner bottom is inscribed with 24 characters in 3 lines. It was collected in 1959.

Preserved in The Palace Museum

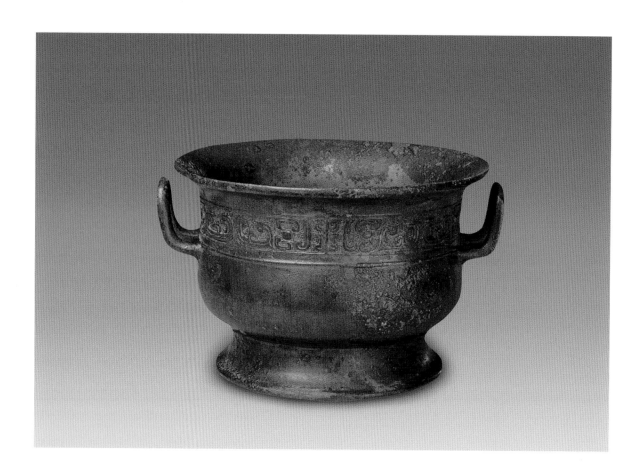

不嬃簋

西周早期

青铜质

宽 33 厘米，通高 15.8 厘米，重 3.14 千克

Gui with Characters Including "嬃"

Early Western Zhou Dynasty

Bronze

Width 33 cm/ Height 15.8 cm/ Weight 3.14 kg

圆腹，侈口，圈足，腹两侧有附耳。口下饰
兽面纹，以云雷纹填地。腹上施一道凸弦纹。
内底铸铭文 24 字。清宫旧藏。

故宫博物院藏

This food vessel has a round belly, a wide
flared mouth, and a ring foot. On each side of
the belly, there is an accessory ear. Below the
rim of the mouth, it is decorated with beast
face patterns with cloud and thunder pattern as
the ground design. There is a streak of convex
string pattern on the belly. The inner bottom is
inscribed with 24 characters. The container was
once preserved in the imperial palace of the
Qing Dynasty.

Preserved in The Palace Museum

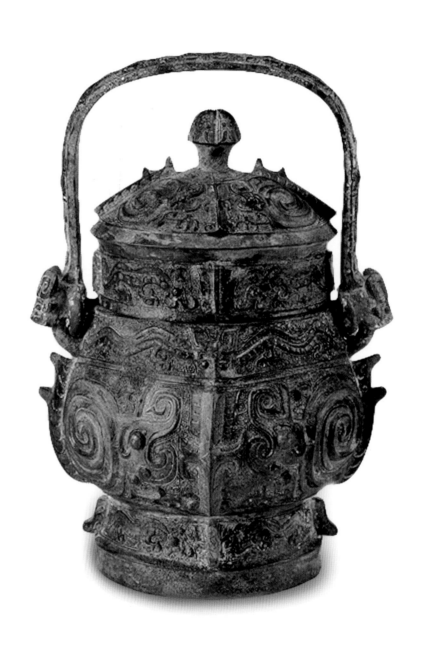

提梁卣

西周早期

青铜质

腹径 15 厘米，高 24 厘米

垂腹，圈足。盖上有钮，提梁两端呈羊首形。
器身饰有蛇纹。古代重要的盛酒器。

泾阳博物馆藏

You with a Looped Handle

Early Western Zhou Dynasty

Bronze

Belly Diameter 15 cm/ Height 24 cm

This vessel has a dropping belly, ring foot, and a knob on the cover. The two ends of the looped handle are in the shape of a sheep' head. It is decorated with snake pattern. It was an important vessel for keeping wine.

Preserved in Jingyang Museum

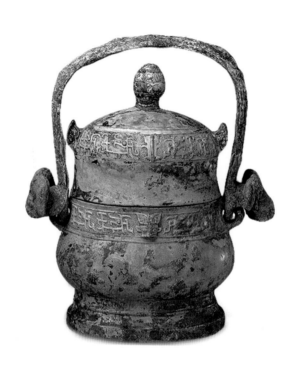

小夫卣

西周早期

青铜质

宽 23.4 厘米，通高 26.5 厘米，重 2.8 千克

You with Characters "Xiao Fu"

Early Shang Dynasty

Bronze

Width 23.4 cm/ Height 26.5 cm/ Weight 2.8 kg

垂腹，圈足。盖钮呈菌状，盖上两侧铸有"犄角"，提梁的两端呈浮雕羊首形。口下及盖沿饰垂冠回首夔龙，以云雷纹填地。提梁饰蝉纹，圈足施弦纹一道。盖内及器底对铭，各铸8字，记小夫为其父丁宗庙做祭器。1958年收购。

故宫博物院藏

This vessel has a drooping belly and a ring foot. There is a knob on the cover of the vessel shaped like a mushroom, and the two sides of the cover are cast with a horn. Both sides of the hoop handle are decorated with a ram head in relief. There are decorations of Kui dragon that turns its head back with its crest dropping downward with cloud and thunder pattern as the ground-tint and cicada patterns on the hoop handle and a streak of patterns on the ring foot. The same inscription of 8 characters is inscribed on the inner side of the cover and the bottom of the vessel. The inscription records that a man named Xiao Fu made sacrificial utensils for his father Ding's temple. It was a acquired in 1958.

Preserved in The Palace Museum

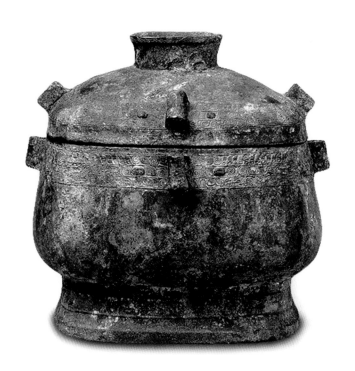

叔卣

西周早期

青铜质

宽 21.6 厘米，通高 19.3 厘米，重 2.82 千克

You with Character "Shu"

Early Shang Dynasty

Bronze

Width 21.6 cm/ Height 19.3 cm/ Weight 2.82 kg

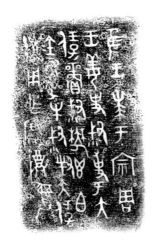

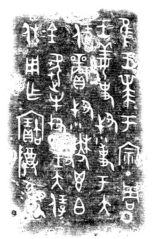

椭方体，方口四角发圆，大腹，圈足。有盖，盖顶呈喇叭形捉手。器颈与盖沿均四面铸有贯耳，两两相对，贯耳是穿系的地方。盖上与器颈部均饰兽面纹带，圈足饰细弦纹两道。卣盖内与器底有对铭，均 5 行 32 字。1959 年由浙江省文物管理委员会调拨。

故宫博物院藏

The vessel has an oval-square body, a large belly, a ring foot, and a square mouth with four rounded corners. The knob on the cover is shaped like a trumpet. On the neck and the edge of the cover there are four opposed tubular ears, where the vessel is tied. There is a belt of animal mask patterns on the cover and the neck, and two streaks of slender string patterns on the ring foot. The inscription on the cover and the bottom is the same, respectively with 32 characters in 5 lines. This vessel was allocated from the Cultural Relics Administration Committee of Zhejiang Province in 1959.

Preserved in The Palace Museum

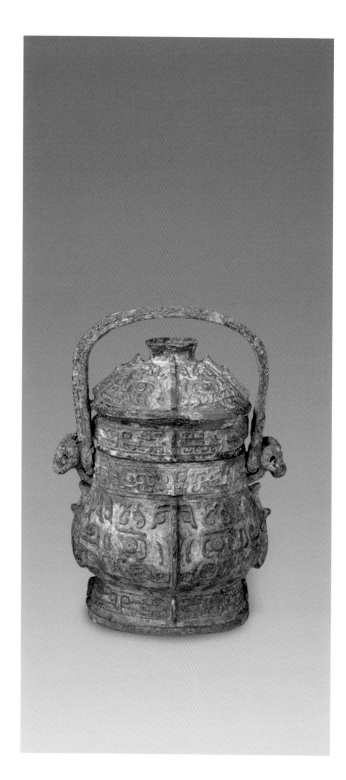

顶卣

西周早期

青铜质

宽 21.3 厘米，通高 27.5 厘米，重 3 千克

You with Character "Ding"

Early Shang Dynasty

Bronze

Width 21.3 cm/ Height 27.5 cm/ Weight 3 kg

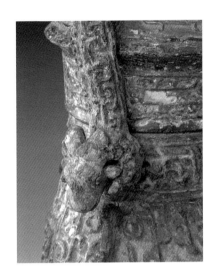

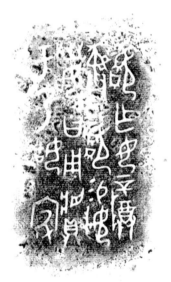

扁圆形器体。盖顶隆起，折沿明显，捉手圈形。器身子母口，鼓腹，圈足有宽边。提梁两端兽首似羊形，面饰蝉纹。盖与器身四面有较宽的扉棱，盖面和器腹饰没有地纹的分解式兽面纹。颈部饰相对回顾式卷尾夔纹，中隔浮雕兽首。盖沿和圈足饰两两相对的四组以分尾夔纹组成的兽面纹。盖内和器底铸铭文 4 行 17 字。1960 年北京市文化局调拨。

故宫博物院藏

The vessel has a flattened circular body. The top of the cover is bulged, with apparent folded edge and a ring knob. The body of the vessel has a snap lid, a swelling belly and a ring foot with a broad edge. The hoop handle is decorated with designs of an animal head on both ends, which are shaped like ram heads, with cicada patterns on there faces. Broad flanges are on the four sides of the cover and the body. There are shredded animal mask patterns without setoff patterns on the surface of the lid and the belly, and opposing Kui dragon patterns with the dragon head turning back and tail rolling up on the neck. The Kui dragon patterns are separated by an animal head in relief. The edge of the cover and the ring foot are decorated with animal mask patterns that consist of four groups of opposing Kui dragon patterns with separated tails. The inscription on the inner side of the cover and on the bottom is simply of 17 characters in 4 lines. This vessel was allocated from Beijing Municipal Bureau of Culture in 1960.

Preserved in The Palace Museum

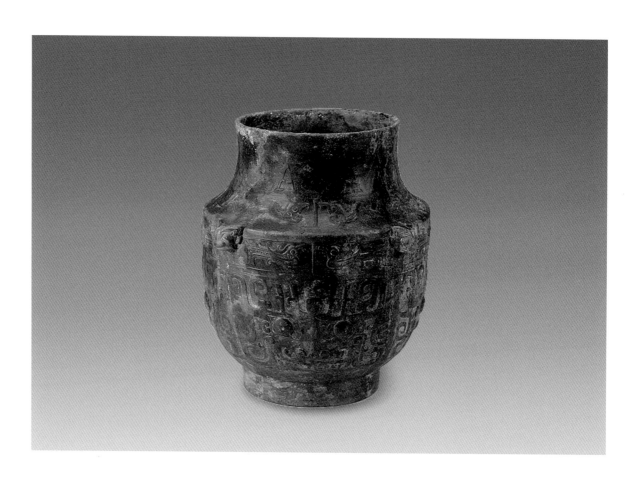

饕餮纹罍

西周早期

青铜质

口径 17 厘米，高 30 厘米

Lei with Tao Tie Pattern

Early Western Zhou Dynasty

Bronze

Mouth Diameter 17 cm/ Height 30 cm

直口，长颈，折肩，深鼓腹，圆底，高圈足，饰饕餮罍纹。罍为容酒器。

泾阳博物馆藏

The vessel has a straight mouth, a long neck, a folded shoulder, a deep swelling belly, a round bottom, and a high ring foot. It has orgre-mask motif and served as a wine vessel. Lei used to serve as a wine vessel.

Preserved in Jingyang Museum

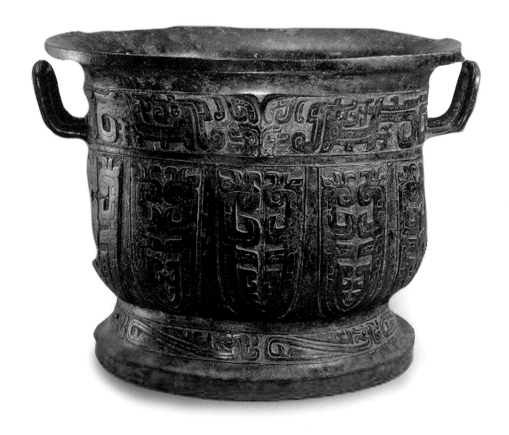

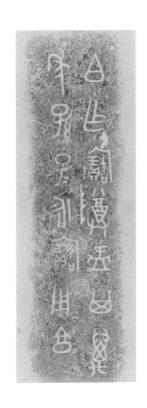

伯盂

西周早期

青铜质

宽 53.3 厘米，通高 39.5 厘米，重 35.8 千克

卷沿，圆腹，二附耳，圈足。颈部前后饰浮雕兽首，兽首两侧饰夔首鸟身的变形夔纹，也称夔鸟纹。腹部饰宽叶纹，圈足上饰对角夔纹。盂内底有铭文 2 行 15 字。清宫旧物 (原藏颐和园)。

故宫博物院藏

Yu with Character "Bo"

Early Western Zhou Dynasty

Bronze

Width 53.3 cm/ Height 39.5 cm/ Weight 35.8 kg

There is a curly edge, round belly, a pair of looped ears, and a ring foot. The neck is decorated with a beast head in relief. On the two sides of the beast head design in relief, there is transformed Kui dragon design, the head of a Kui dragon and the tail of a bird, also called Kui-bird design. The belly is decorated with wide leaf-like pattern, and the ring foot is decorated with diagonally dragon design. The inner bottom is inscribed with 15 characters in 2 lines. It was an antique from the imperial palace of the Qing Dynasty (originally kept in the Summer Palace).

Preserved in The Palace Museum

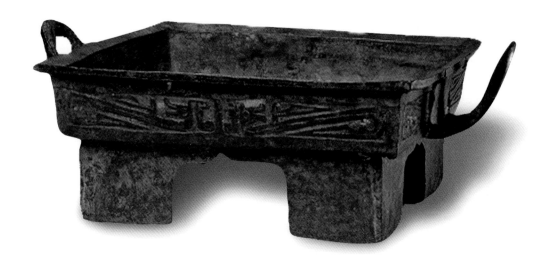

束方盘

西周早期

青铜质

宽 41.5 厘米，通高 14.9 厘米，重 6.82 千克

Square Plate with Character "Shu"

Early Western Zhou Dynasty

Bronze

Width 41.5 cm/ Height 14.9 cm/ Weight 6.82 kg

长方体，浅腹，直壁，平底，宽口沿外折，双附耳。足呈直角形，四个足组成矩形，腹饰卷身夔纹。铭文"束"字位于盘内壁上。1946年入藏。

故宫博物院藏

The cuboid plate has a shallow belly, straight walls, a flat bottom, a wide mouth with edges folded outward, a pair of looped ears, and four right-angled feet forming a rectangle. The belly is decorated with curly Kui dragon design. There is a character "shu" inscribed on the inner wall of the plate. It was collected in 1946.

Preserved in The Palace Museum

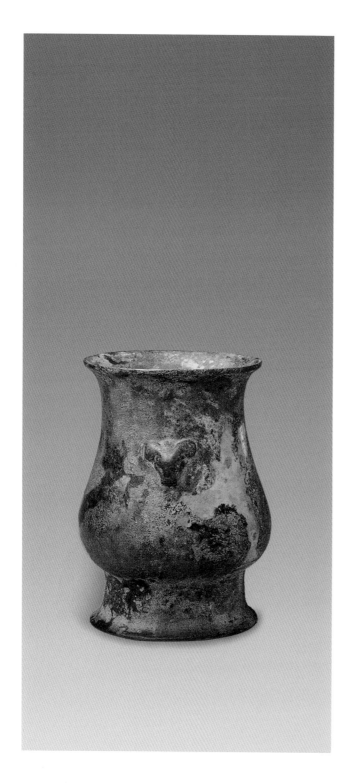

齐史疑觯

西周早期

青铜质

口径 6.6~8 厘米，通高 11.2 厘米，重 0.24 千克

Zhi with Characters "Qi Shi Yi"

Early Western Zhou Dynasty

Bronze

Calibre 6.6-8 cm/ Height 11.2 cm/ Weight 0.24 kg

侈口，宽颈，腹下垂较深，圈足。器外饰有
2 个羊首。器底铸 2 行 8 字铭文，记齐的史
官疑为其祖父辛做的这件宝彝。河南洛阳出
土，1958 年收购。

故宫博物院藏

This drinking vessel has a wide mouth, a wide
neck, a deep drooping belly, and a ring foot.
There are two sheep-head sculptures on the
outer wall. There are 8 characters in 2 lines
inscribed on the bottom, recording that it was
made by a historiographer of the Qi State as
a present for his grandfather. The vessel was
unearthed in Luoyang City, Henan Provence. It
was acquired collected in 1958.

Preserved in The Palace Museum

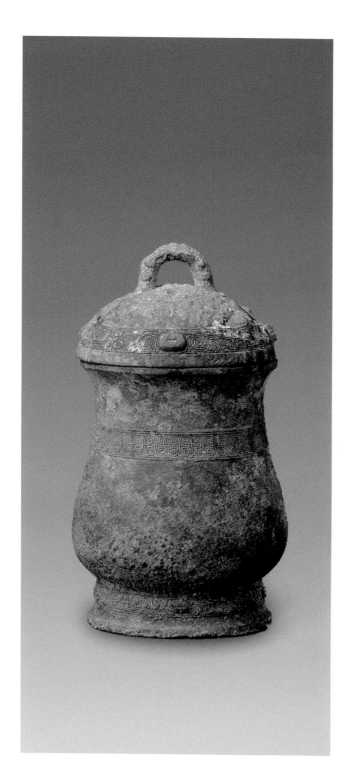

疑觯

西周早期

青铜质

宽 8.9 厘米，通高 15.4 厘米，重 0.54 千克

Zhi with Character "Yi"

Early Western Zhou Dynasty

Bronze

Width 8.9 cm/ Height 15.4 cm/ Weight 0.54 kg

敞口，束颈，下腹向外倾垂，圈足外侈。有盖，盖呈弧面，钮呈半环状。盖沿及圈足饰目雷纹，器颈部饰云雷纹。盖和器均有铭文6字，记疑做宝尊彝。1961年收购。

故宫博物院藏

This drinking vessel has a wide mouth, a convergent neck, a belly whose lower part droops outward, a ring foot, a cover with a cambered surface, and a semi-ring knob. The edge of the cover and the ring foot are decorated with eye-like designs and the neck is decorated with cloud and thunder pattern. 6 characters are inscribed on both of the cover and the vessel body. It was acquired in 1961.

Preserved in The Palace Museum

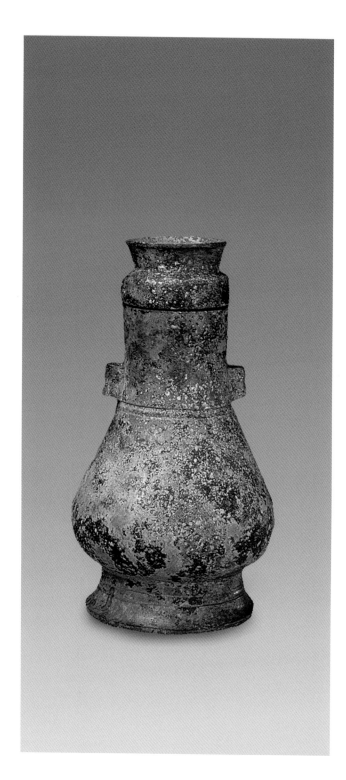

保侃母壶

西周早期

青铜质

口径 9.3 厘米，通高 31.4 厘米，重 2.9 千克

Pot with Characters "Bao Kan Mu"

Early Western Zhou Dynasty

Bronze

Mouth Diameter 9.3 cm/ Height 31.4 cm/

Weight 2.9 kg

口圆，颈略短，两侧有贯耳，腹庞大，圈足，有盖。颈、足各饰一道弦纹。盖内与器底对铭，各铸有铭文 3 行 14 字。记王后赏赐其女官宝侃母贝，为答谢王后的美意，特做此壶。1955 年 12 月收购。

故宫博物院藏

The pot has a round mouth, a relatively short neck, a tubular ear on both sides of the large belly, and a ring foot. The pot has its own cover. The vessel neck and the ring foot are respectively decorated with a belt string pattern. The inner part of the cover and the vessel bottom has an inscription of 14 characters in 3 lines. The content of the inscription is about a female official named Bao Kan Mu Bei making this pot for the very purpose of showing her gratitude for the queen's award. It was collected in December 1955.

Preserved in The Palace Museum

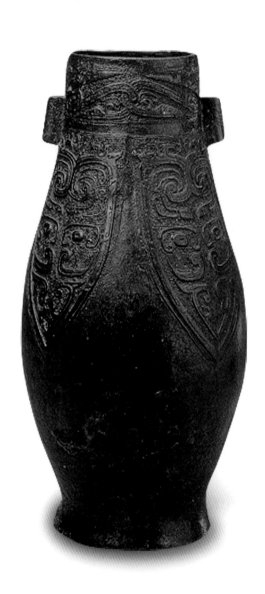

劋妳壶

西周早期

青铜质

口径 9 厘米，通高 31.4 厘米，重 2.35 千克

长颈，两侧有贯耳，深腹，中部渐鼓而下收，圈足随下腹壁成弧状外撇。

口沿处饰有一道虺纹，下饰兽面纹。口内铸有 2 行 5 字铭文，记劋妳自做宝壶。清宫旧物（原藏颐和园）。

故宫博物院藏

Bronze Pot with Characters Including "劋"

Early Western Zhou Dynasty

Bronze

Mouth Diameter 9 cm/ Height 31.4 cm/ Weight 2.35 kg

The pot has a long neck, a tubular ear on both side of the body, a deep belly with a gradually swelling mid-section and a tapered lower-section. The ring foot turns slightly outward in a curved shape along with the lower belly. The rim of the mouth is decorated with snake pattern, and the lower section with design of beast face. Inside the vessel mouth there is an inscription of 5 characters in 2 lines. The content of the inscription is about who making this precious pot. The utensil was an antique from the imperial palace of the Qing Dynasty (originally stored in the Summer Palace).

Preserved in The Palace Museum

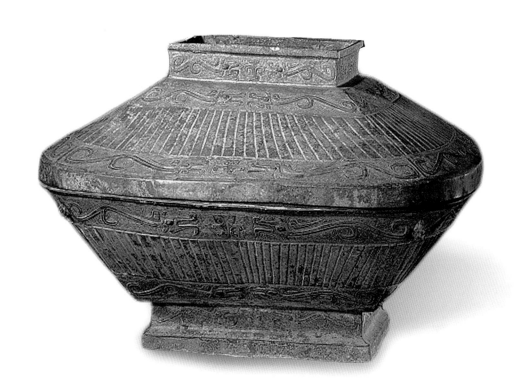

夔纹方器

西周早期

青铜质

宽 55.8 厘米，通高 37 厘米，重 17.5 千克

Square Vessel with Kui Dragon Designs

Early Western Zhou Dynasty

Bronze

Width 55.8 cm/ Height 37 cm/ Weight 17.5 kg

器呈长方形，四角发圆。深腹，侈口，自口沿向下收敛，使器身形成斜直的斗状。足呈矩形，足底宽，足腰稍内凹。有盖，盖与器的大小基本相同，亦作斜坡状，盖顶有长方形捉手，可以"却置"，即合上为一器，打开则为相同的两器。全器上下饰有花纹，器颈与腹下部、盖沿与盖上部、矩形足与捉手四面均饰夔纹。器和盖上的夔纹装饰手法相同，长身，眼凸起，张口，一角，一足，卷尾，并都以云雷纹为衬托。器腹与盖上的主题纹饰是直线纹，直线呈辐射状分布，形成了与器形相统一的风格。1957 年国家文物局调拨。

故宫博物院藏

The vessel is in a rectangular shape with four rounded corners. It has a deep belly and a large mouth which tapers itself downward from the mouth of the vessel, making the vessel like an oblique and straight "dou" (a vessel with four sides that droop downward and convergently). The foot is in rectangular shape with broad margin and indent waist. The cover and the mouth of the vessel are roughly the same in size, and the four sides of the cover are shaped in slope form. There is a rectangle handle on the top of the cover which has the function of switching itself from one piece to two pieces of vessel or vice versa. The whole vessel is decorated with decorative patterns: with the same technique of carving the Kui dragon pattern on the neck and the lower belly of the vessel: long body, protruding eyes, one horn, one foot, curling tail, all of which take square cloud and thunder pattern as the ground-tint, The theme pattern on the belly and the cover is primarily in straight lines, radiating to different directions and echoing the style of the body shape. It was allocated from State Administration of Cultural Heritage in 1957.

Preserved in The Palace Museum

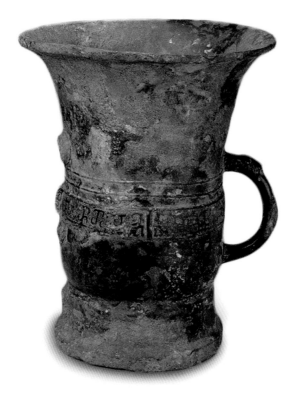

盠司土幽尊

西周早期

青铜质

宽 18 厘米，通高 21 厘米，重 1.78 千克

Zun with Characters "Zhou Si Tu You"

Early Western Zhou Dynasty

Bronze

Width 18 cm/ Height 21 cm/ Weight 1.78 kg

侈口，深腹，圈足。腹一侧有兽首錾，十分独特。腹上部饰云雷纹衬底的夔纹一周。内底铸铭文 2 行 9 字。1956 年收购。

故宫博物院藏

The vessel has a flared mouth, a deep belly, and a ring foot. On one side of the body of the vessel, there is a unique handle shaped like beast head. The upper belly is decorated with a circle of Kui dragon pattern with cloud and thunder pattern as ground-tint. The bottom inside the vessel is inscribed with 9 characters in 2 lines. The vessel was acquired in 1956.

Preserved in The Palace Museum

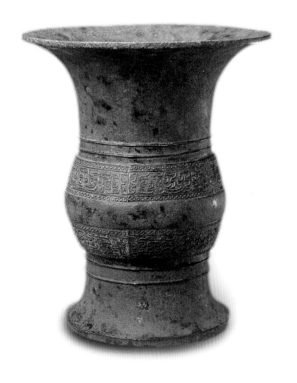

微师耳尊

西周早期

青铜质

宽 23.2 厘米，通高 25.7 厘米，重 3.48 千克

Zun with Characters "Wei Shi Er"

Early Western Zhou Dynasty

Bronze

Width 23.2 cm/ Height 25.7 cm/ Weight 3.48 kg

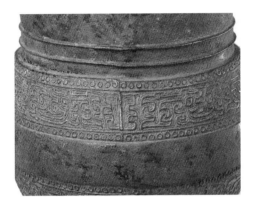

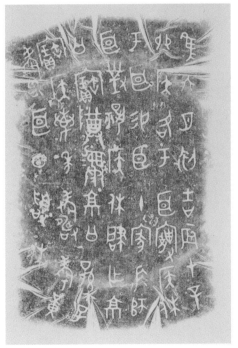

圆筒形，侈口，鼓腹，圈足。颈下与圈足上部均饰弦纹两道。腹部上下两周纹带均饰以双线勾勒的变形夔纹，夔纹带上下用圈带纹镶边。尊内底有铭文7行52字。1961年国家文物局调拨。

故宫博物院藏

The vessel has a barrel-like body, a flared mouth, a swelling belly, and a ring foot. The lower neck and upper foot are both decorated with two circles of bowstring patterns. The upper and lower sections of the belly are decorated with transformed Kui dragon designs outlined with double lines and edged with circles in belt-like pattern. On the inner bottom, there is an inscription of 52 characters in 7 lines. The vessel was allocated from State Administration of Cultural Heritage in 1961.

Preserved in The Palace Museum

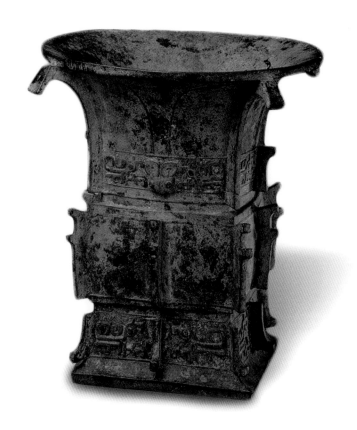

觳父乙方尊

西周早期

青铜质

口径 20.5 厘米，通高 23 厘米，重 3.52 千克

Square Zun with Characters Including "觳"

Early Western Zhou Dynasty

Bronze

Mouth Diameter 20.5 cm/ Height 23 cm/ Weight 3.52 kg

形体粗壮，口、颈皆圆，方腹，方圈足。有觚棱，饰夔纹。内底有铭文 3 行 15 字，大意为其父乙宗庙中的祭器宝彝，子孙后代永宝用。1958 年收购。

故宫博物院藏

The vessel has a large body, a round mouth and neck, a square belly, and a square ring foot. There are square ridges decorated with Kui dragon pattern. The inner bottom of the vessel is inscribed with 15 characters in 3 lines, recording that this wine vessel was made as a sacrificial utensil used in a ancestral temple for his father and the vessel should be treated was made as a permanent treasure and used by the descendants. The relic was acquired in 1958. Preserved in The Palace Museum

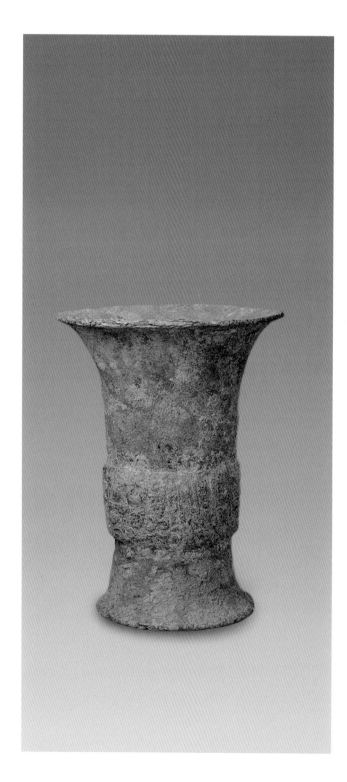

古伯尊

西周早期

青铜质

宽 22.1 厘米，通高 27.4 厘米，重 2.5 千克

Zun with Characters "Gu Bo"

Early Western Zhou Dynasty

Bronze

Width 22.1 cm/ Height 27.4 cm/ Weight 2.5 kg

敞口，鼓腹，高圈足。腹部饰兽面纹。这是
商代晚期到西周早期流行的三段式筒状尊。
内底有铭文 32 字。1956 年收购。

故宫博物院藏

The vessel has a large mouth, a swelling belly,
and a tall ring foot. The belly is decorated with
beast face pattern. The three-part barrel-like
vessel represents a popular style of wine vessels
from Late Shang Dynasty to early Western
Zhou Dynasty. There is an inscription of 32
characters on the bottom of the vessel. The relic
was acquired in 1956.

Preserved in The Palace Museum

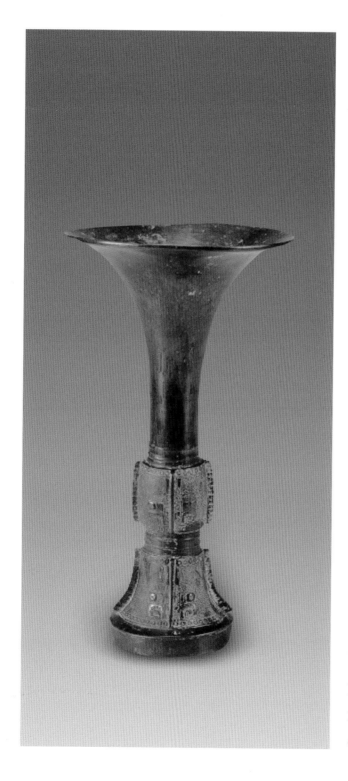

觚

西周早期

青铜质

口径 16.4 厘米，高 28.8 厘米

Gu

Early Western Zhou Dynasty

Bronze

Calibre 16.4 cm/ Height 28.8 cm

喇叭口，细腰，高圈足，分成三部分，饰四
道扉棱。饮酒器。

泾阳博物馆

The container a trumpet-like mouth, a slender
waist, a high ring foot. It is divided into three
parts decorated with four leaf ridge. It served as
a wine-drinking vessel.

Preserved in Jingyang Museum

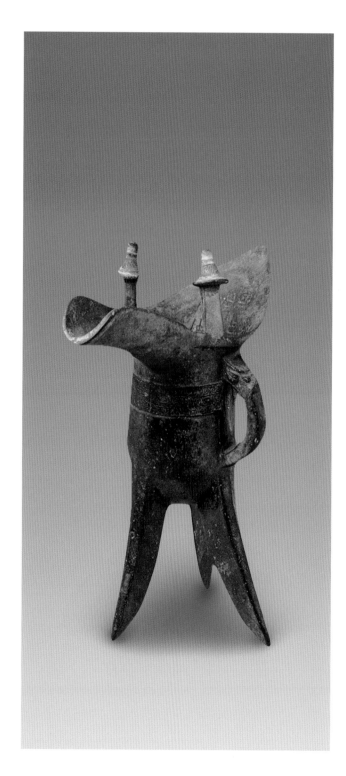

和爵

西周早期

青铜质

口径 17.8 厘米，通高 21.3 厘米，重 0.98 千克

Jue with Character "He"

Early Western Zhou Dynasty

Bronze

Calibre 17.8 cm/ Height 21.3 cm/ Weight 0.98 kg

长颈，深腹，鋬小而粗，圜底，刀形足外侈。菌状双柱较高，立于口沿近流处，腹饰兽面纹。口内有 3 行 9 字铭文，记和为其做召伯的父亲做宝尊彝。1958 年收购。

故宫博物院藏

The vessel has a long neck, a deep belly, a small and thick handle, a round bottom, and blade-shaped tripodal deet which all stretch outward. There are two relatively high fungus-shaped pillars standing on the edge of the mouth near the spout. The belly is decorated with beast face pattern. There is an inscription of 9 characters in 3 lines on the inner side of the mouth, recording that the vessel was made by He who made "Bao Zun Yi"(a sacrificial vessel) for his father whose official position was Zhao Bo. It was acquired in 1958.

Preserved in The Palace Museum

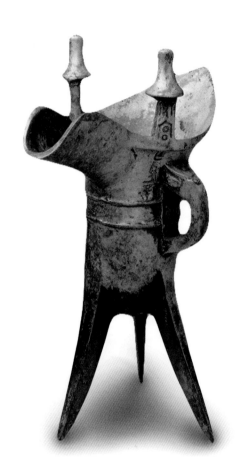

守宫父辛爵

西周早期

青铜质

宽 16.2 厘米，通高 22.7 厘米，重 0.76 千克

Jue with Characters "Shou Gong Fu Xin"

Early Western Zhou Dynasty

Bronze

Width 16.2 cm/ Height 22.7 cm/ Weight 0.76 kg

宽流，帽形长柱，鋬上端雕铸兽头，中腰微
收，下承三个宽形刀状足。腹施两道弦纹。
柱上下铭文 5 字，记守宫为父辛做器。1964
年入藏。

故宫博物院藏

The vessel has a wide spout, with two long cap-shaped pillars. An animal head is carved on the top of the handle. The waistline is slightly concave. On the lower part of the vessel, there are wide blade-shaped tripodal feet. Two circles of string patterns are carved on the belly. There is an inscription of 5 characters, recording that the vessel was made by Shou Gong for his father Xin. It was collected in 1964.

Preserved in The Palace Museum

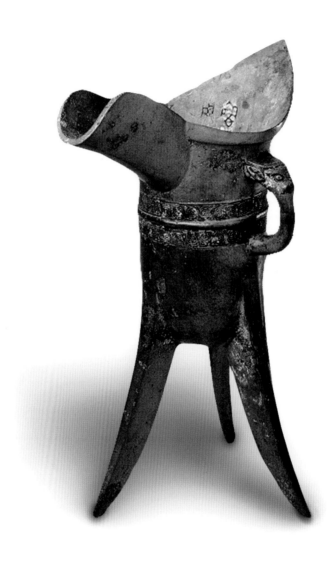

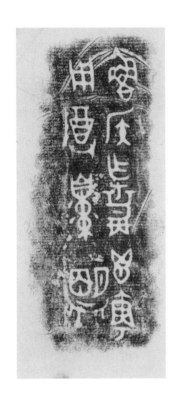

鲁侯爵

西周早期

青铜质

宽 16.2 厘米，通高 20 厘米，重 0.76 千克

爵体略长而优美，流尾上翘，爵壁较直，无柱。鋬较小，饰有兽首。圆底，刀形足外撇。腹上下二层云雷纹带，中间隔以突起的弦纹。尾部口壁内铸有 2 行 10 字铭文，是爵中铭文较长者。1962 年国家文物局调拨。

故宫博物院藏

Jue with Characters "Lu Hou"

Early Western Zhou Dynasty

Bronze

Width 16.2 cm/ Height 20 cm/ Weight 0.76 kg

The whole body is slightly long and elegant. The tail of the spout turns up, and the walls of the vessel are straight. There are no pillars. The handle is smaller than normal ones on which there is a beast head design. The vessel has a round bottom, and blade-shaped tripodal feet that stretch outward. There are two layers of cloud and thunder patterns on lower and upper parts of the the belly, which are separated by a bulgy bowstring pattern. There is an inscription of 10 characters in 2 lines on the inner side of the the tail wall. The inscription is comparatively longer than others. It was allocated from the State Administration of Cultural Heritage.

Preserved in The Palace Museum

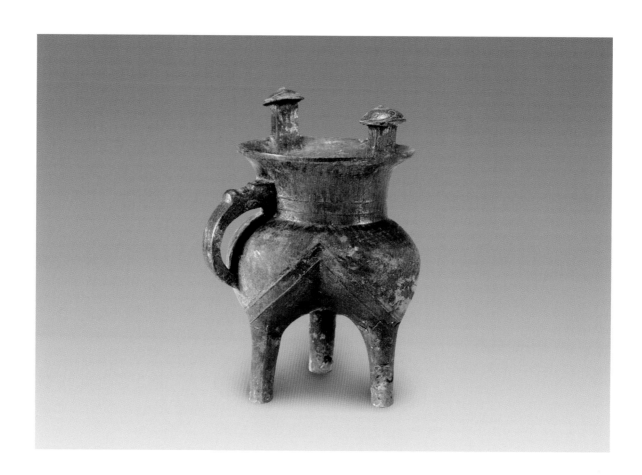

弦纹斝

西周早期

青铜质

口径 18 厘米，通高 30 厘米

Jia with Bowstring Pattern

Early West Zhou Dynasty

Bronze

Diameter 18 cm/ Height 30 cm

三足一錾，敞口束腰，下腹部骤然外鼓，与
上腹部于腰际形成明显折棱，柱形足。腰部
和腹部各饰两道弦纹。

泾阳博物馆藏

This is three-footed vessel with a handle, and
it has a flared mouth and a convergent waist.
The lower part of the belly protrudes outward,
creating a folded ridge at the waist. The feet are
columnar, and two streaks of bowstring pattern
are decorated on the waist and the belly.

Preserved in Jingyang Museum

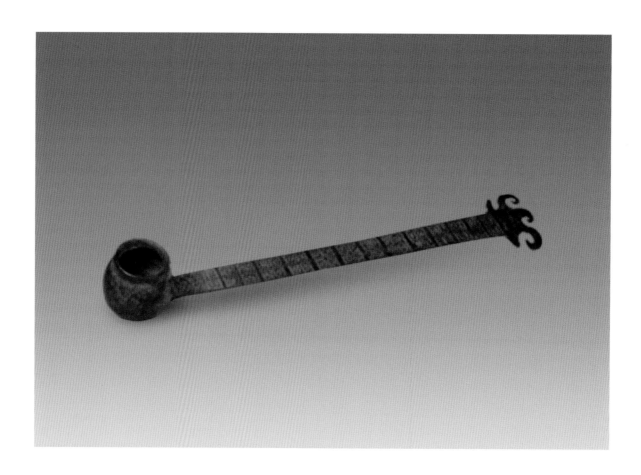

雷纹柄勺

西周早期

青铜质

通长 41.7 厘米，斗高 5.5 厘米，重 0.46 千克

Ladle with a Handle with Thunder Pattern

Early Zhou Dynasty

Bronze

Length 41.7 cm / Bucket Height 5.5 cm/ Weight 0.46 kg

圆口，圜底，直柄，后尾云端为透雕。柄上饰规整的雷纹。勺通常被用来挹取酒浆。1962 年收购。

故宫博物院藏

The bowl of this ladle has both a round bottom and a round mouth. The ladle has a straight handle with a hollowed-out sculpture at the end. This handle is decorated with evenly spaced thunder patterns. The vessel was commonly utilized for ladling wine liquids. It was acquired in 1962.

Preserved in The Palace Museum

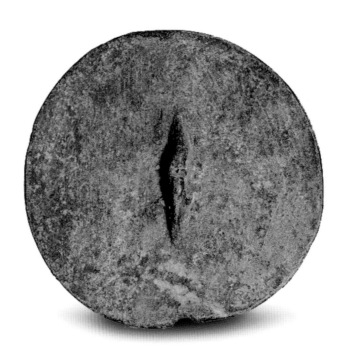

素镜

西周早期

铜质

直径 6.5 厘米

Plain Mirror

Early Western Zhou Dynasty

Copper

Diameter 6.5 cm

桥形钮，无钮座，通体光素无纹，是西周时期罕见的铜镜之一。1958 年陕西宝鸡市郊出土。

宝鸡青铜器博物院藏

The mirror has a bridge-like knob without pedestal. The mirror is smooth and has no decorative patterns. It is one of the rare bronze mirrors in Western Zhou Dynasty ever discovered. It was excavated in the suburbs of Baoji City, Shaanxi Province, 1958.

Preserved in Baoji Bronze Ware Museum

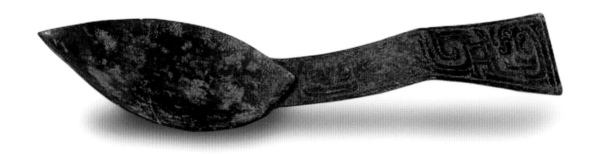

夔纹匕

西周早期

青铜质

宽 5.6 厘米，通高 23.4 厘米，重 0.2 千克

体呈桃叶状，后有扁条柄，上饰夔纹。1964 年收购。

故宫博物院藏

Bi with Kui Dragon Pattern

Early Western Zhou Dynasty

Bronze

Width 5.6 cm/ Height 23.4 cm/ Weight 0.2 kg

This vessel is in the shape of a peach leaf. The back part is a flat long handle decorated with Kui dragon patterns. It was acquired in 1964.

Preserved in The Palace Museum

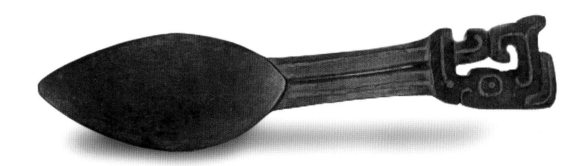

窃曲纹匕

西周中期

青铜质

宽 3.9 厘米，通高 17.8 厘米，重 0.12 千克

桃叶形体，扁条柄，柄末端饰透雕窃曲纹。1959 年收购。

故宫博物院藏

Bi with Qie Qu Pattern

Middle Western Zhou Dynasty

Bronze

Width 3.9 cm/ Height 17.8 cm/ Weight 0.12 kg

This type of ancient spoons is in the shape of a peach leaf. It has a flat long handle whose end part is hollow

engraved with Qie Qu pattern. It was acquired in 1959.

Preserved in The Palace Museum

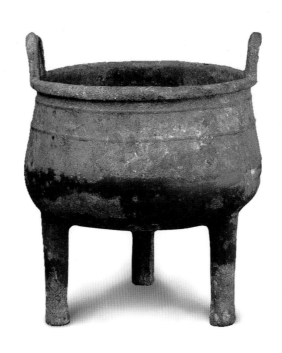

𦭒鼎

西周中期

青铜质

宽 18.6 厘米，通高 21.2 厘米，重 2.04 千克

Tripod with Character "𦭒"

Mid Western Zhou Dynasty

Bronze

Width 18.6 cm/ Height 21.2 cm/ Weight 2.04 kg

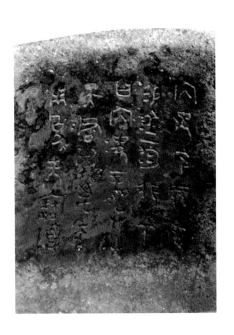
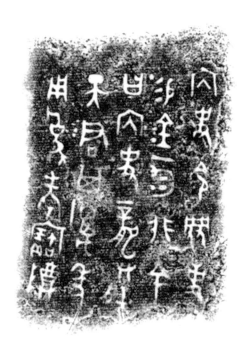

圆腹，折沿，二立绳耳，三柱足。口下饰弦纹二道。鼎内有铭文 5 行 26 字。

故宫博物院藏

The tripod has a round belly, a folded edge, two prick twisted-rope-type ears, and three columnar legs. Under the rim of the mouth on the outside, there are two streaks of string pattern. There is a 26-character inscription in 5 lines inside the tripod.

Preserved in The Palace Museum

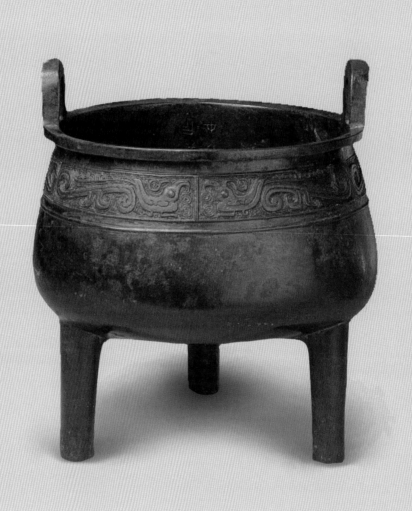

才僤父鼎

西周中期

青铜质

宽 19.8 厘米，通高 22 厘米，重 2.72 千克

立耳，柱足，下腹向外倾垂。口下饰分尾长鸟纹，细云纹填地。内壁铸铭文记才僤父自做尊彝。清宫旧藏。

故宫博物院藏

Tripod with Characters Including "僤"

Mid Western Zhou Dynasty

Bronze

Width 19.8 cm/ Height 22 cm/ Weight 2.72 kg

The tripod has prick ears and columnar legs. The lower part of the belly leans outward. The area under the rim of the mouth on the outside is decorated with long bird pattern with separated tails, and the fine cloud designs are used as the ground pattern. There is an inscription on the inner wall of the tripod, recording that a man made this vessel. The tripod belongs to the collection of the imperial palace of the Qing Dynasty.

Preserved in The Palace Museum

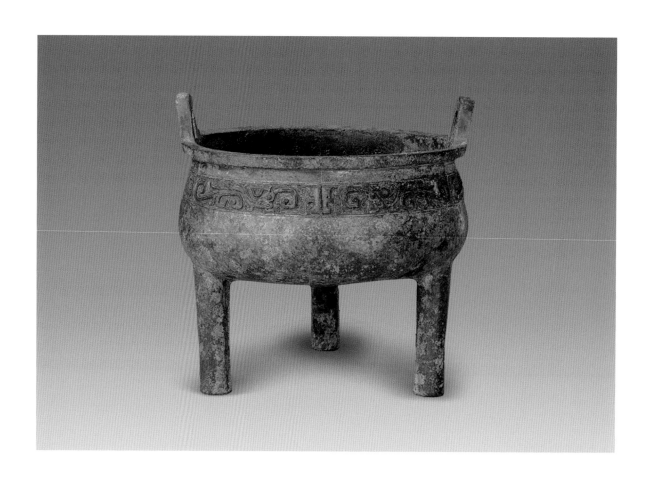

师旂鼎

西周中期

青铜质

宽 17.6 厘米，通高 15.8 厘米，重 1.92 千克

Tripod with Characters "Shi Qi"

Mid Western Zhou Dynasty

Bronze

Width 17.6 cm/ Height 15.8 cm/ Weight 1.92 kg

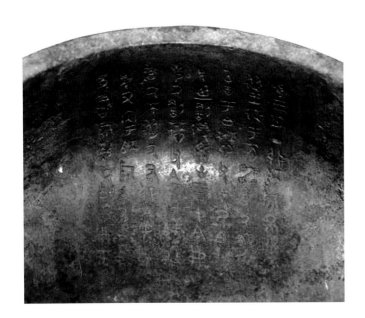
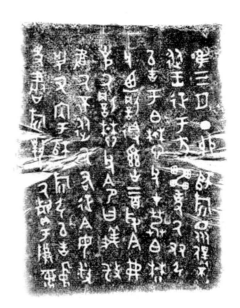

圆浅腹，腹部稍倾垂，三柱足，二直耳。口沿下饰一周长身、分尾、垂喙的鸟纹，以云雷纹为衬托。鼎内壁铸铭文 8 行 79 字。1955 年国家文物局调拨。

故宫博物院藏

The tripod has a shallow round belly that leans slightly outward, three columnar legs, and two prick ears. Below the rim of the mouth on the outside, there is a circle of designs of a bird with a long body, a separated tail, and a hanging beak; the cloud and thunder patterns are used as a foil to them. On the inner wall, there is a 79-character inscription in 8 lines. The tripod was allocated from State Administration of Cultural Heritage in 1955.

Preserved in The Palace Museum

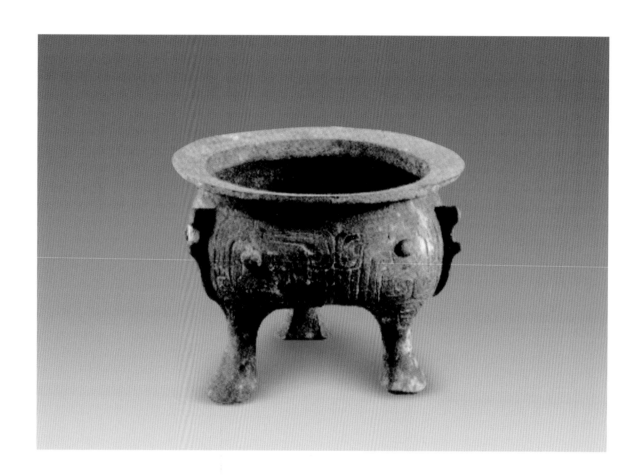

中枏父鬲

西周中期（前 950—前 850)

青铜质

口径 19.5 厘米，高 14 厘米

Li with Characters "Zhong Nan Fu"

Mid Western Zhou Dynasty (950 B.C.–850 B.C.)

Bronze

Mouth Diameter 19.5 cm/ Height 14 cm

鬲在商周时期是烹煮食品的器具，兼具灶和锅的功能，并为重要的礼器，作为国家重要活动的象征而存在。此件造型别致，古朴大气。口沿及内腹壁铸有 38 字的短文，记载了其主人中枏父的一些生平事迹，是已发现的铜鬲铭文中最长的，具有重要的史料价值。

陕西历史博物馆藏

During the Shang and Zhou Dynasties, "Li" was used as a utensil for cooking, serving the roles of both the hearth and the pan. It also served as an important sacrificial vessel and the symbol of important national activities. This cooking vessel has a unique style with pristine beauty and elegance. There is an inscription of 38 words on the edge and the inner wall of the belly, recording the life story of its owner. This cooking vessel has the longest inscription among the discovered bronze "Li" vessels. It is of great value in historical research.

Preserved in Shaanxi History Museum

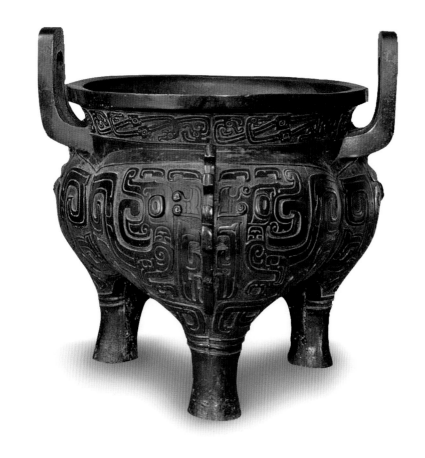

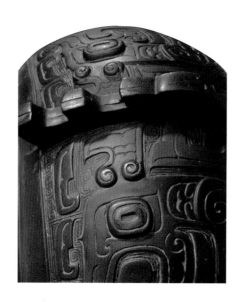

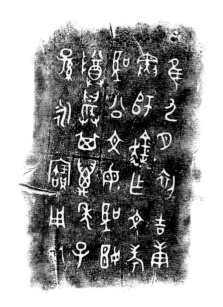

师趛鬲

西周中期

青铜质

宽 54.6 厘米，通高 50.8 厘米，重 48.8 千克

师趛鬲是迄今所知鬲中最大且最华丽的一件。本器表面经打磨上蜡，颜色黑中透亮，极精致、美观。全器纹饰由三种纹样组成：腹部以云雷纹为地，上以凸雕的六只巨大回首夔纹为主体纹饰；颈部饰双首夔龙回曲纹带；附耳内、外两侧均饰以重环纹。器腹内壁铸有铭文 5 行 29 字。1955 年从上海收购。

故宫博物院藏

Li with Characters "Shi Yin"

Mid Western Zhou Dynasty

Bronze

Width 54.6 cm/ Height 50.8 cm/ Weight 48.8 kg

Up to now, Li with characters "Shi Yin" is the largest and the most magnificent one among all the known Li vessels. With polishing and waxing on the surface, brightness of this vessel is expressed from its dark color. This cooking vessel is of extreme delicacy and beauty. There are three patterns on this cooking vessel. On the belly, the protruded pattern of six huge Kui dragons turning their heads is chosen as the main pattern, with Yun-lei (cloud-thunder) pattern being used as setoff; the curved pattern of double-headed Kui dragon which looks like the Chinese character "回" is decorated on the neck; multiple layers of ring patterns are decorated inside and outside the accessory ears. On the inner wall of the belly, there is a 5-line inscription of 29 words. The cooking vessel was acquired in Shanghai in 1955.

Preserved in The Palace Museum

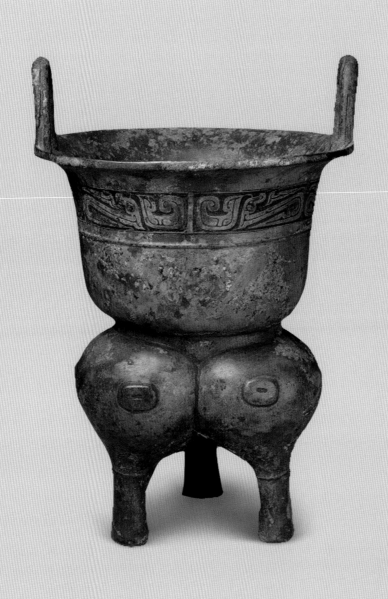

孚公甗

西周中期

青铜质

宽 31.3 厘米，通高 43.5 厘米，重 7.47 千克

甑、鬲合体。甑呈深圆形，侈口，立耳，腹微敛；鬲部分裆，裆缝连于腰际，三足正向蹄形发展。颈部饰回首垂冠的夔鸟纹，足上部饰粗犷的兽面纹。铭文 2 行 9 字。1952 年收购。

故宫博物院藏

Yan with Characters "Fu Gong"

Mid Western Zhou Dynasty

Bronze

Width 31.3 cm/ Height 43.5 cm/ Weight 7.47 kg

The cooking vessel is a combination of Zeng steamer caldron and Li cooking vessel. The deep round Zeng has a flared mouth, two prick ears, and a convergent belly. The tripod has a separated crotch that is connected with the waist. The three feet are hoof-shaped. The neck is decorated with transformed Kui dragon pattern, and the Kui lowers its crest and turns its head back. The upper part of the feet is decorated with boorish patterns of beast face. There is an inscription of 9 characters in 2 lines. It was acquired in 1952.

Preserved in The Palace Museum

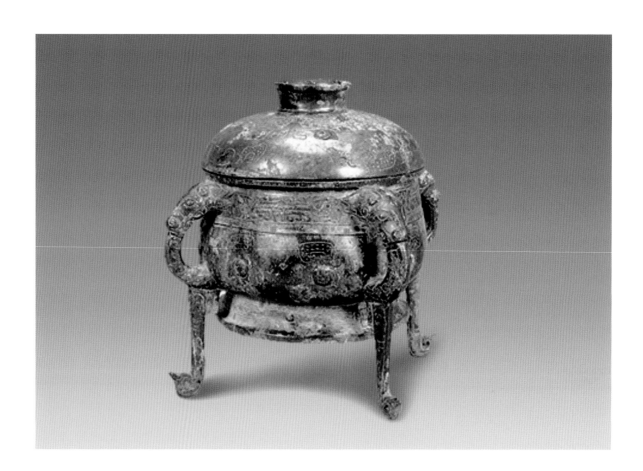

青铜四足簋

西周中期（前 950—前 850）

青铜质

腹径 19.9 厘米，高 25 厘米，足高 9.3 厘米

Four Legged Bronze Gui

Mid Western Zhou Dynasty (950 B.C.–850 B.C.)

Bronze

Belly Diameter 19.9 cm/ Height 25 cm/ Height of the Leg 9.3 cm

此件结构较为复杂，装饰技巧独特。腹内底部和盖的内壁上均有"白(伯)乍(作)簋"3字铭文。其中的簋字，左边是一个有底足的盛有食品的器皿，右边是一支持有器具的手，这是我们断定簋为食器的依据之一。山西省曲沃县曲村晋国墓地出土。

北京大学赛克勒考古与艺术博物馆藏

This food vessel is sophisticated in structure and unique in decoration technique. The inner bottom of the belly and the inner side of the cover are both inscribed with the three characters "Bo Zuo Gui". For the character "Gui", it is written in two parts: the left side is a vessel with a foot that has food in it; the right side is a hand that holds a ware. This is one of the evidences that we determine that Gui is a food utensil. It was unearthed in the graveyard of Jin State in history, which is located in Qu Village, Quwo County, Shanxi Province.
Preserved in Arthur M. Sackler Museum of Art and Archaeology at Peking University

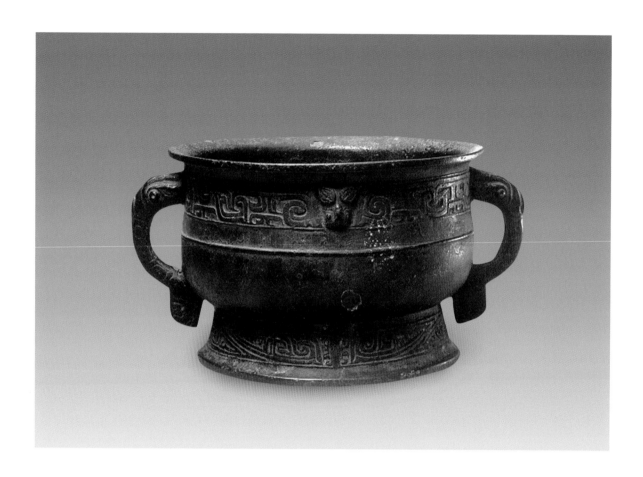

筥小子簋

西周中期

青铜质

宽 28.4 厘米，通高 14.3 厘米，重 2.94 千克

Gui with Characters "Ju Xiao Zi"

Mid Western Zhou Dynasty

Bronze

Width 28.4 cm/ Height 14.3 cm/ Weight 2.94 kg

侈口，束颈，鼓腹。两首兽耳，垂珥较短。矮圈足有宽边。口沿下两侧均以突起的小兽首为中心，饰相对称的窃曲纹带。圈足饰斜角云纹。器内底铸铭文 25 字。1956 年冯公度先生家属捐献。

故宫博物院藏

The food vessel has a wide flared mouth, a convergent neck, a swelling belly, a pair of accessory handles shaped like beast head on each side of the belly with short dropping decoration, and a short ring foot with a wide rim. Under the rim of the mouth, the two sides of the vessel take the protuberant animal head as the center, and are decorated with belts of ragged curve. The ring foot is decorated with oblique cloud pattern. The inner bottom is inscribed with 25 characters. It was donated by the family of Mr. Feng Gongdu in 1956.

Preserved in The Palace Museum

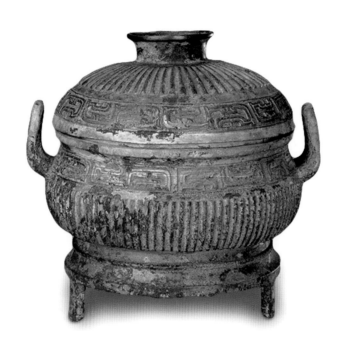

甂簋

西周中期

青铜质

宽 23.8 厘米，通高 21.1 厘米，重 3.96 千克

Gui with Character "Cui"

Mid Western Zhou Dynasty

Bronze

Width 23.8 cm/ Height 21.1 cm/ Weight 3.96 kg

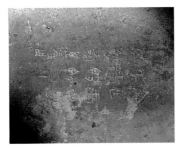

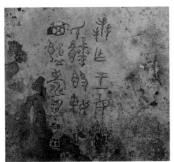

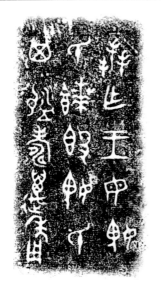

圆形，鼓腹，侈口，折沿，有二附耳，有盖，盖顶有圆形捉手，圈足下附三矮足。器颈与盖沿各饰一周窃曲纹带，腹与盖均饰直道纹，圈足上饰粗弦纹一道。簋盖、器对铭，3 行 16 字。河南洛阳出土，1957 年国家文物局调拨。

故宫博物院藏

The round food container has a plump belly with two looped ears, a wide flared mouth, folded edge and a cover. On the top of the cover, there is a knob handle. Below the ring foot are three short feet. The neck of the container and the edge of the cover are both decorated with a circle of ragged curve belts. The belly and the cover are both decorated with the design of streak pattern, and the ring foot is decorated with a streak of thick string pattern. The cover and the body part of the container are inscribed with 16 characters in 3 lines. It was unearthed from Luoyang City, Henan Province. This vessel was allocated from State Administration of Cultural Heritage in 1957.

Preserved in The Palace Museum

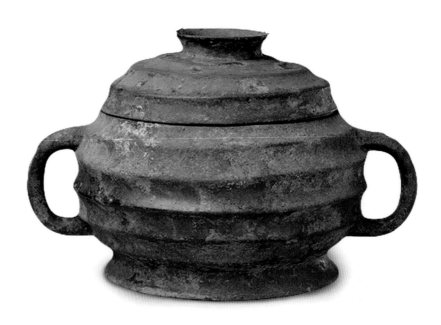

敔簋

西周中期

青铜质

宽 29.2 厘米，通高 17.8 厘米，重 3.18 千克

Gui with Character "敔"

Mid Western Zhou Dynasty

Bronze

Width 29.2 cm/ Height 17.8 cm/ Weight 3.18 kg

敛口，有盖，器腹向外倾垂甚扁，圈足外侈，体侧有半环状耳一对。此簋盖、器均饰横向瓦楞文。盖内与器底铸有相同的铭文 28 字。1954 年收购。

故宫博物院藏

The container has a convergent mouth and a cover. With its belly extending outward and downward, it forms a relatively oblate shape. The ring foot extends outward. On each side of the belly, there is a pair of ears in half ring. Both the cover and the body are decorated with horizontal tile-ridge pattern. The inner side of the cover and the bottom of the container are inscribed with the same 28 characters. It was acquired in 1954.

Preserved in The Palace Museum

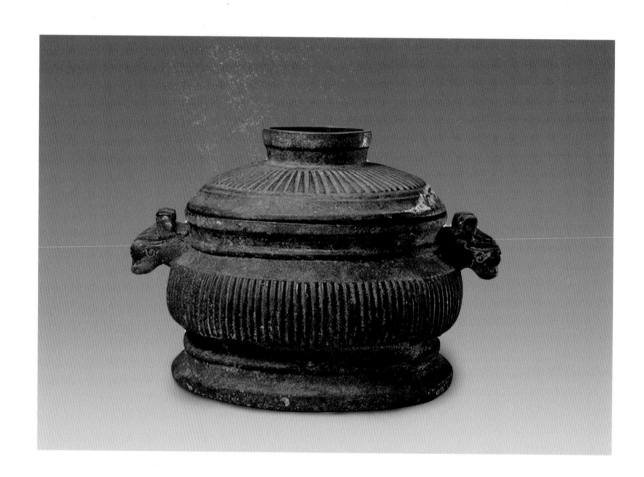

太师虘簋

西周中期

青铜质

宽 30.2 厘米，通高 20.7 厘米，重 6.12 千克

Gui with Characters "Tai Shi Cuo"

Mid Western Zhou Dynasty

Bronze

Width 30.2 cm/ Height 20.7 cm/ Weight 6.12 kg

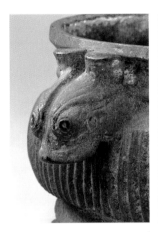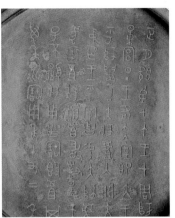

矮体，鼓腹，圈足。器颈两侧有风格独特的兽头錾。有盖，盖顶捉手呈喇叭形。盖面与器腹均饰竖直纹，器颈及圈足上各饰粗弦纹一道。簋盖内和器底各铸铭文 7 行 70 字。传于 1941 年陕西西安出土，国家文物局调拨。

故宫博物院藏

The food container has a short body, a swelling belly, and a ring foot. On each side of the neck are two uniquely designed handles in the shape of beast heads. On the top of the cover is the trumpet-like knob handle. Both the surface of the cover and the belly of the container are decorated with the pattern of vertical straight lines. The neck and the ring foot are decorated with thick string patterns, respectively. The inner side of the cover and the bottom of the container are inscribed with 70 characters in 7 lines respectively. It's said that the container was unearthed in Xi'an in 1941. This vessel was allocated from State Administration of Cultural Heritage.

Preserved in The Palace Museum

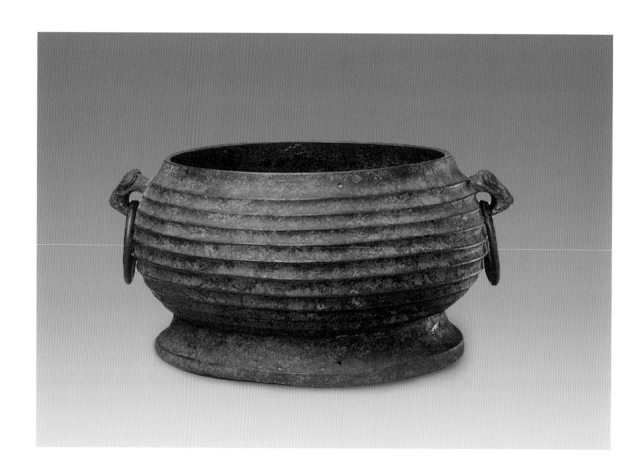

豆闭簋

西周中期

青铜质

宽 32.5 厘米，通高 15.1 厘米，重 5.06 千克

Gui with Characters "Dou Bi"

Mid Western Zhou Dynasty

Bronze

Width 32.5 cm/ Height 15.1 cm/ Weight 5.06 kg

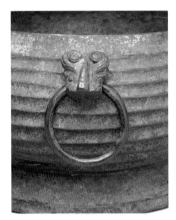 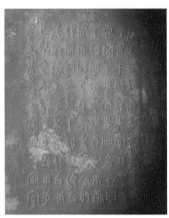 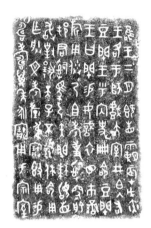

圆鼓腹，弇口，圈足。腹两侧有兽首衔环耳，
器身自上而下满饰平行的瓦楞文。簋内底铸
铭文 9 行 92 字。1957 年收购。

故宫博物院藏

The food container has a round swelling belly,
a small mouth, and a ring foot. On each side of
the belly are two handles in the shape of beast
heads holding loops in their mouth. The body
is fully decorated with horizontal tile ridge-like
patterns from top to bottom. The inner side of
the bottom is inscribed with 92 characters in
9 lines. It was acquired in 1959.
Preserved in The Palace Museum

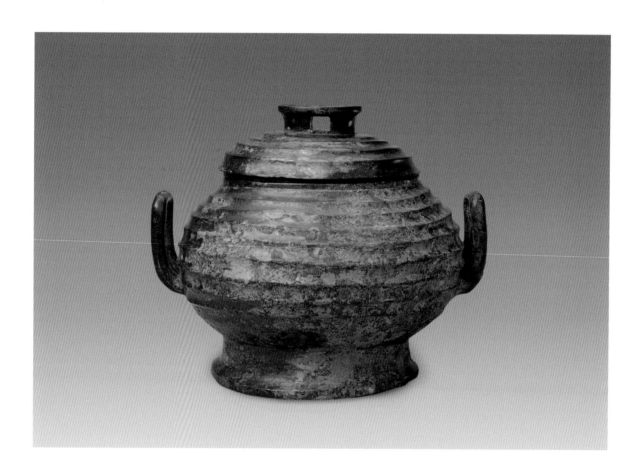

綪簋

西周中期

青铜质

宽 24.5 厘米，通高 19.2 厘米，重 3.14 千克

Gui with Character "綪"

Mid Western Zhou Dynasty

Bronze

Width 24.5 cm/ Height 19.2 cm/ Weight 3.14 kg

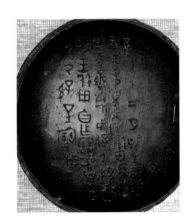

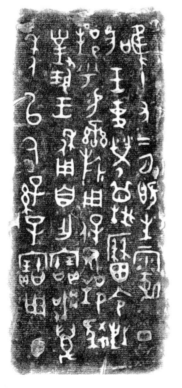

敛口，鼓腹，器与盖有子母口相合，盖上捉手呈圈状，器腹两侧有附耳一对，圈足较低。此簋通身饰瓦楞文。盖、器对铭，均有44字。1958年收购。

故宫博物院藏

The food container has a convergent mouth and a swelling belly. There is a snap-lid with a knob on the top in the form of rings. On each side of the belly is a pair of looped ears. The ring foot is relatively short, and the whole container is decorated with tile ridge-like patterns. The cover and the body are inscribed with 44 characters respectively. It was acquired in 1958.

Preserved in The Palace Museum

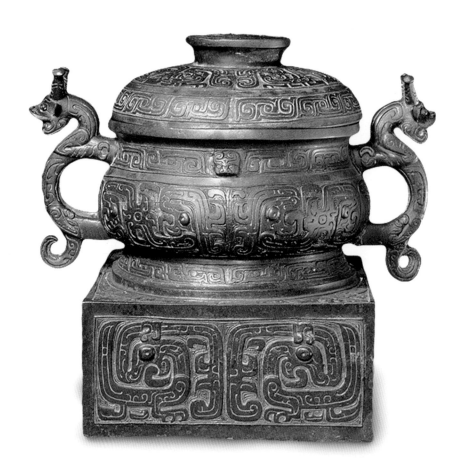

追簋

西周中期

青铜质

宽 44.5 厘米，通高 38.6 厘米，重 18.9 千克

器体较大，隆盖，顶有圆形捉手，侈口，鼓腹，圈足，下附方座。腹部两侧以回顾形龙为耳。盖缘、口沿下饰窃曲纹，腹部饰连体龙纹，方座饰卷体龙纹。盖、器同铭，各铸 7 行 60 字。盛食器。清宫旧物（原藏颐和园）。

故宫博物院藏

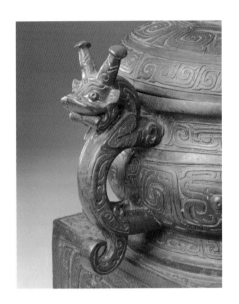

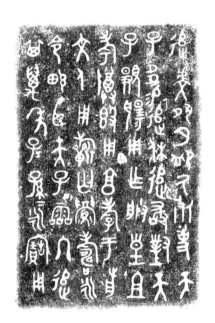

Gui with Character "Zhui"

Mid Western Zhou Dynasty

Bronze

Width 44.5 cm/ Height 38.6 cm/ Weight 18.9 kg

This huge food container has a wide flared mouth, a swelling belly, a ring foot, and a hunched cover with a knob handle on the top. There is a square pedestal at the bottom of the vessel. On each side of the belly is a pair of handles shaped like dragons that look back. The lower part of the cover edge and the areas below the rim of the mouth are decorated with ragged curve. The belly is decorated with siamesed dragon patterns, and the square pedestal is decorated with the pattern of curled-up dragons. The inscriptions on the cover and the body of the vessel are the same, both with 60 characters respectively in 7 lines. It was an antique of the imperial palace of the Qing Dynasty (originally kept in the Summer Palace).

Preserved in The Palace Museum

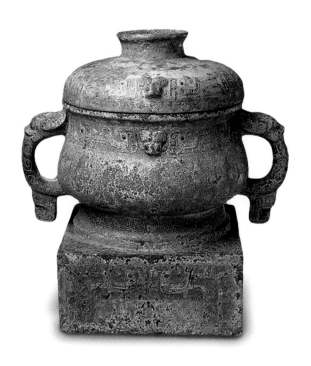

滕虎簋

西周中期

青铜质

宽 31.7 厘米，通高 33.6 厘米，重 7.4 千克

Gui with Characters "Teng Hu"

Mid Western Zhou Dynasty

Bronze

Width 31.7 cm/ Height 33.6 cm/ Weight 7.4 kg

侈口，深腹，兽耳有珥，圈足下连铸方座。有盖，盖的捉手呈圈状，颈和盖沿还增饰浮雕兽头。圈足上饰目雷纹。盖、器同铭，有3行14字，记滕虎为其父亲公命仲做祭祀宝彝。清宫旧物（原藏颐和园）。

故宫博物院藏

This vessel has a wide flared mouth, a deep belly, a pair of handles with design of a beast head and decoration, and a ring foot supported by a square pedestal. There is a knob shaped like rings on the cover. The neck and the cover edge are decorated with beast heads in relief. The ring foot is decorated with the eye-like patterns intertwined with squared whorled (thunder) designs. Both the cover and the body of the vessel are inscribed with the same 14 characters in 3 lines to record that a man named "Teng Hu" cast this precious vessel to make sacrifices for his father. It was an antique of the timperial palace of the Qing Dynasty (originally kept in the Summer Palace).

Preserved in The Palace Museum

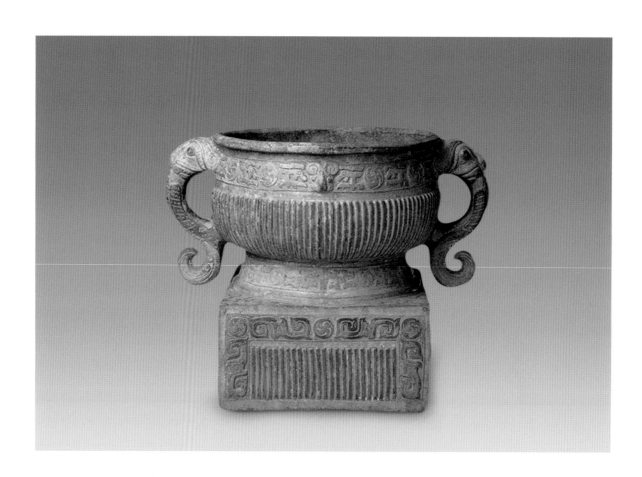

格伯簋

西周中期

青铜质

宽 30.8 厘米，通高 23.5 厘米，重 7.58 千克

Gui with Characters "Ge Bo"

Mid Western Zhou Dynasty

Bronze

Width 30.8 cm/ Height 23.5 cm/ Weight 7.58 kg

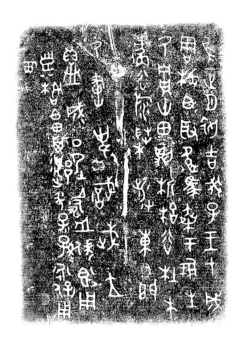

圆腹，圈足，下有方座。二兽头耳，耳下端似象鼻卷曲。器颈前、后正中各铸一凸起的兽头，兽头两侧饰夔纹和圆涡纹。腹部和方座四壁中心饰竖直纹。圈足饰连续的四瓣花和圆涡纹带。方座四壁边缘饰圆涡纹和窃曲纹，方座顶部四角饰兽面纹。簋内底有铭文8行83字。1958年收购。

故宫博物院藏

This vessel has a round belly and a ring foot with a square pedestal at the bottom. There is a pair of handles in the shape of beast heads on each side of the belly. The lower end of the handle is like a curled elephant nose. The center of both the front and back sides of the neck are respectively cast with a beast head in relief, and the two sides of the beast heads are decorated with Kui dragon pattern and vortex pattern. The belly and the centers of the walls of the pedestal are decorated with vertical streak lines. The ring foot is decorated with successive four-petal flower designs and round vortex pattern. The edges of the walls of the square pedestal are decorated with round vortex pattern and ragged curve. The top four corners of the square pedestal are decorated with beast face patterns. There is an inscription of 83 characters in 8 lines on the inner side of the bottom of the vessel. It was acquired in1958.

Preserved in The Palace Museum

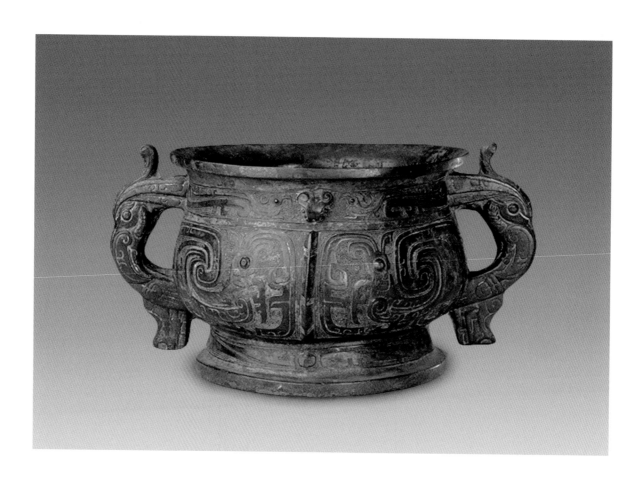

伯作簋

西周中期

青铜质

宽 29.2 厘米，通高 14.9 厘米，重 2.4 千克

Gui with Characters "Bo Zuo"

Mid Western Zhou Dynasty

Bronze

Width 29.2 cm/ Height 14.9 cm/ Weight 2.4 kg

矮体，垂腹，束颈，侈唇。通身以云雷纹作地，满饰不同姿态的凤鸟。颈部为分尾长鸟纹，中隔浮雕兽头；腹部呈垂冠分尾大凤鸟，两两对峙，形象优美。器内底铭文"伯作簋"3字。清宫旧藏。

故宫博物院藏

This vessel has a short body, a dropping belly, a convergent neck and a large lip. The whole body has cloud and thunder patterns as the ground over which birds in different postures are designed. The neck part is decorated with the pattern of a bird with long body and a divided tail. An embossment of animal head separates the belly in the middle. The belly is decorated with big phoenixes with lowered crest and divided tails, and they are in a face-to-face posture on both sides of the body, and appear exquisite and beautiful. There is an inscription of 3 characters of "Bo Zuo Gui" on the inner bottom of the vessel. This item is an antique from the imperial palace of the Qing Dynasty. Preserved in The Palace Museum

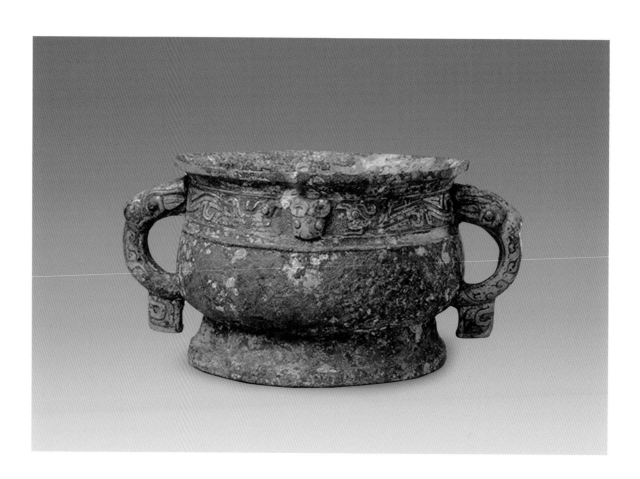

朢簋

西周中期

青铜质

宽 27 厘米，通高 13.2 厘米，重 2.2 千克

Gui with Character "朢"

Mid Western Zhou Dynasty

Bronze

Width 27 cm/ Height 13.2 cm/ Weight 2.2 kg

圆鼓腹，侈口，束颈，圈足，双兽耳。颈部
饰鸟纹带，鸟垂喙、长卷尾，两两相对，鸟
纹间加饰小兽首。簋内底有铭文 5 行 40 字。
1961 年国家文物局调拨。

故宫博物院藏

This vessel has a wide flared mouth, a round
swelling belly, a convergent neck, and a ring
foot. There is a pair of handles in the shape of
beast heads. The neck is decorated with a band
of the pattern of birds with a dropping beak, and
a long curled tail, and a face-to-face posture.
Within the bird patterns there are decorations
of small beast heads. The inner bottom of the
container is inscribed with 40 characters in
5 lines. This vessel was allocated from State
Administration of Cultural Heritage in 1961.
Preserved in The Palace Museum

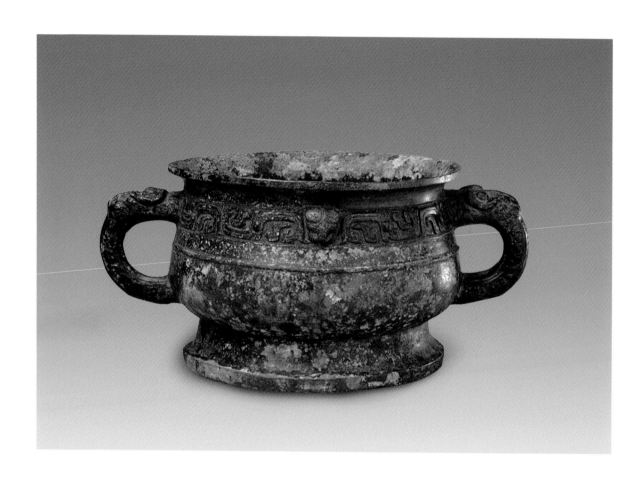

同簋

西周中期

青铜质

宽 32.3 厘米，通高 14.2 厘米，重 3.9 千克

Gui with Character "Tong"

Mid Western Zhou Dynasty

Bronze

Width 32.3 cm/ Height 14.2 cm/ Weight 3.9 kg

圆形，侈口，鼓腹，圈足，双兽首耳。颈部前、后对称雕铸兽头，兽头两侧是窃曲纹带；腹部有一道凸弦纹。盖、器同铭。1956 年收购。

故宫博物院藏

This round vessel has a wide flared mouth, a swelling belly, a ring foot, and a pair of handles in the shape of beast heads. The neck is symmetrically decorated with the design of beast heads on both the front and back sides. Along the two sides of the beast heads there is a decoration of ragged curve. There is a streak of convex string pattern on the belly. Both the cover and the body of the vessel are inscribed with the same characters. It was acquired in 1956.

Preserved in The Palace Museum

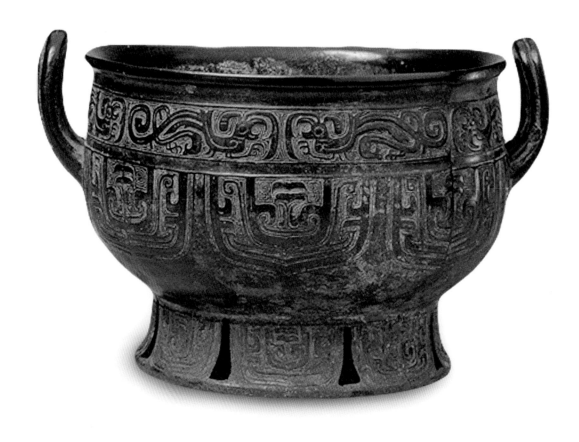

鸟纹簋

西周中期

青铜质

宽 24.4 厘米，通高 15.9 厘米，重 2.22 千克

深圆腹，侈口，圈足较矮，腹两侧有附耳。颈部饰凤鸟纹，高冠长尾，造型舒展不拘；腹上与圈足均施宽叶纹。此簋的形制和装饰都较为特殊。1946 年入藏。

故宫博物院藏

Gui with Bird Pattern

Mid Western Zhou Dynasty

Bronze

Width 24.4 cm/ Height 15.9 cm/ Weight 2.22 kg

The vessel has a deep round belly, a wide flared mouth, and a short ring foot. There is a pair of looped handles on each side of the belly. The neck is decorated with phoenixes of a high crest and a long tail that are free in posture. Both the belly and the ring foot are decorated with the pattern of wide leaves. The appearance and the decoration of this vessel are quite unique. It was collected in 1946.

Preserved in The Palace Museum

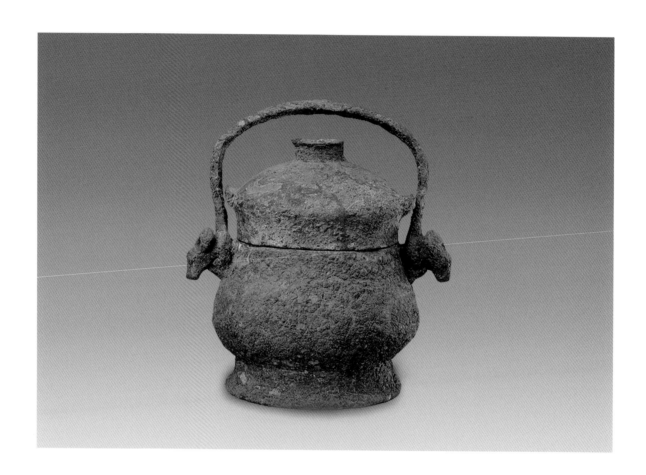

作册虤卣

西周中期

青铜质

宽 21.7 厘米，通高 23.4 厘米，重 2.58 千克

You with Characters Including "虤"

Mid Shang Dynasty

Bronze

Width 21.7 cm/ Height 23.4 cm/ Weight 2.58 kg

盖有捉手，左、右出现直立的"犄角"。提
梁两端呈兔首形。腹下部膨出，圈足。卣盖、
器对铭，6 行 63 字。河南洛阳出土，1961
年国家文物局调拨。

故宫博物院藏

The cover of this vessel has a knob and a horn
on both the right and the left sides. The two
ends of the hoop handle are shaped into a rabbit
head. The lower part of the belly is swelling.
There is a ring foot. The same inscription of 63
characters in 6 lines is made on both the cover
and the body of the vessel. It was excavated
in Luoyang City, Henan Province, and was
allocated from State Administration of Cultural
Heritage in 1961.

Preserved in The Palace Museum

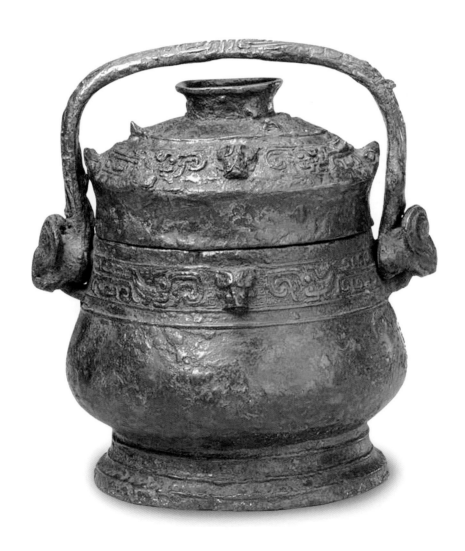

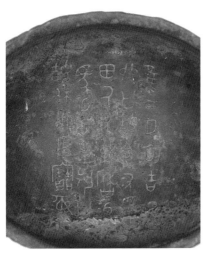

次卣

西周中期

青铜质

宽 21.5 厘米，通高 21.8 厘米，重 2.44 千克

圆鼓腹，圈足。有盖，盖顶有喇叭形握，盖两侧铸直立的"犄角"。器以半环衔接提梁，提梁两端雕饰兽头。器颈与盖前、后均铸有浮雕兽首，兽首两侧饰鸟纹带。卣盖、器同铭，均 5 行 30 字。1958 年收购。

故宫博物院藏

You with Character "Ci"

Mid Shang Dynasty

Bronze

Width 21.5 cm/ Height 21.8 cm/ Weight 2.44 kg

This vessel has a swelling belly, a ring foot, a cover with a trumpet-shaped knob with an upright horn on both sides of the cover. For this vessel, there is a hoop handle with both ends decorated with an animal head design and connected with the body of the vessel by an half-ring. Both on the front and back of the cover and the neck, an animal head design in relief is made with a belt of bird pattern cast on its right and left sides. The cover and the body have the same inscription of 30 characters in 5 lines. The vessel was acquired in 1958.

Preserved in The Palace Museum

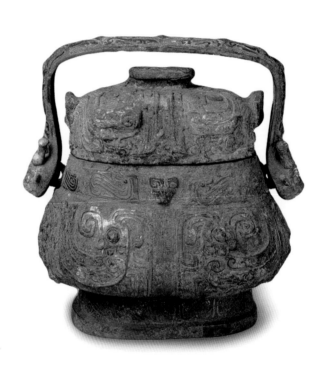

夺卣

西周中期

青铜质

口径 18.5~19.8 厘米，通高 27.5 厘米，重 2.07 千克

You with Character "Duo"

Mid Shang Dynasty

Bronze

Mouth Diameter 18.5–19.8 cm/ Height 27.5 cm/ Weight 2.07 kg

椭圆体，腹外鼓，下垂很低，有提梁，圈足。有盖，盖沿不折边，呈圆顶的帽状，圆形捉手。周身通饰鸟纹。盖、器对铭，各 2 行 9 字，记夺为其父丁做宝尊彝。1954 年国家文物局调拨。

故宫博物院藏

This oval vessel has a swelling belly, a hoop handle, and a ring foot and the belly droops to a very low position. The cover is shaped like a vaulted hat with a round knob and an unfolded edge. The whole body of the vessel is decorated with bird patterns. There is an inscription of 9 characters in 2 lines both on the cover and the body of the vessel, which records that Duo made this treasured vessel for his father. The vessel was allocated from State Administration of Cultural Heritage in 1954.

Preserved in The Palace Museum

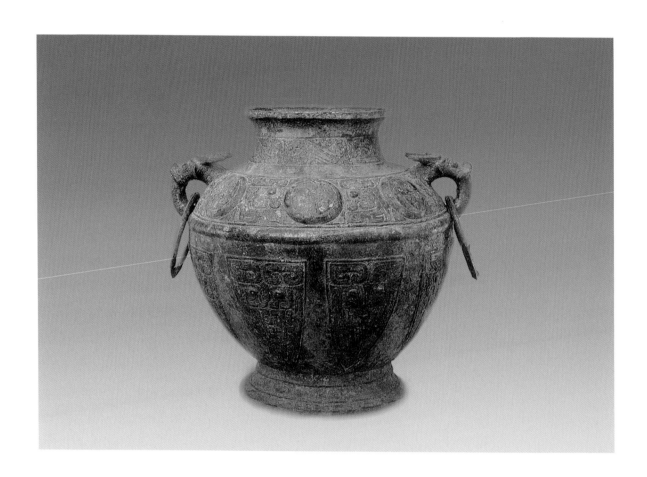

洀御史罍

西周中期

青铜质

宽 36 厘米，通高 33.3 厘米，重 9.9 千克

Lei with Characters "Yan Yu Shi"

Mid Western Zhou Dynasty

Bronze

Width 36 cm/ Height 33.3 cm/ Weight 9.9 kg

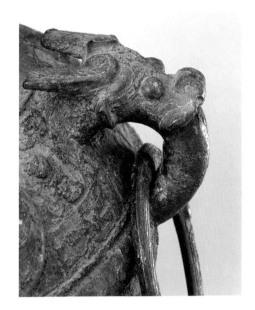

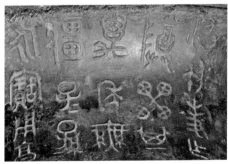

平沿，斜肩，肩上有兽首衔环双耳，腹斜收。颈饰窃曲纹，肩饰涡纹间变体夔纹，腹饰蕉叶对夔纹。口内铭文5行19字。1956年冯公度先生家属捐献。

故宫博物院藏

The mouth of the vessel has a flat edge, an oblique shoulder with two ears in the shape of a head of a sacred animal holding a ring, and a belly that collects obliquely. The neck is decorated with successive ragged curve, the shoulder with vortex pattern intertwined with transformed Kui dragon pattern, and the belly with banana leaf pattern facing the Kui dragon pattern. There is an inscription of 19 characters in 5 lines on the inner rim of the mouth. This vessel was donated in 1956 by family members of Mr.Feng Gongdu.

Preserved in The Palace Museum

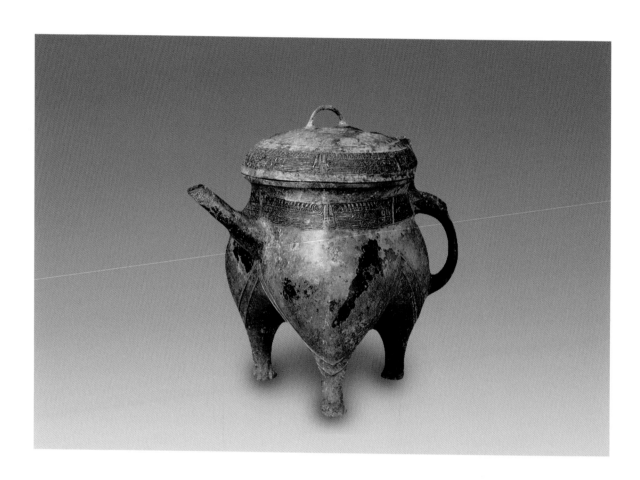

来父盉

西周中期

青铜质

口径 13.5 厘米，通高 21.5 厘米，重 2.14 千克

He with Characters "Lai Fu"

Mid Western Zhou Dynasty

Bronze

Caliber 13.5 cm/ Height 21.5 cm/ Weight 2.14 kg

口边沿外翻，束颈，肩略广，鋬与盖相套铸，袋腹不甚深，下具三柱足。盖及口下各饰有兽面纹和弦纹，足饰二道弦纹。盖、器对铭，各有铭文2行10字，器铭于鋬旁。1958年收购。

故宫博物院藏

The edge of the mouth is extended outward. The neck is straight. The shoulder is big. The handle and the cover are designed to join each other. The belly is not very deep, with three cylindrical legs below. On the cover and below the mouth, there is beast face pattern and bowstring pattern. On the legs, there are two lines of bowstring pattern. There is an inscription of 10 characters in 2 lines both on the cover and the vessel body. The inscription on the body of the vessel is beside the handle. It was acquired in 1958.

Preserved in The Palace Museum

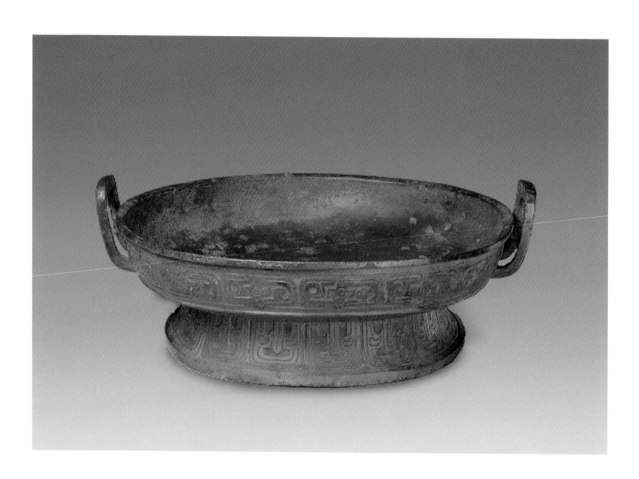

殷毃盘

西周中期

青铜质

宽 39.6 厘米，通高 13.7 厘米，重 4.57 千克

Plate with Characters Including "毃"

Mid Western Zhou Dynasty

Bronze

Width 39.6 cm/ Height 13.7 cm/ Weight 4.57 kg

圈足，双附耳。腹饰窃曲纹，圈足饰垂叶纹，均用方雷纹填地。器内底铸铭文 18 字。1946 年入藏。

故宫博物院藏

There is a ring foot with leaf-like design, a pair of looped ears, and a belly decorated with Qie Qu patterns. All these designs take thunder pattern as the ground-tint. 18 characters are inscribed on the inner bottom. The plate was collected in 1946.

Preserved in The Palace Museum

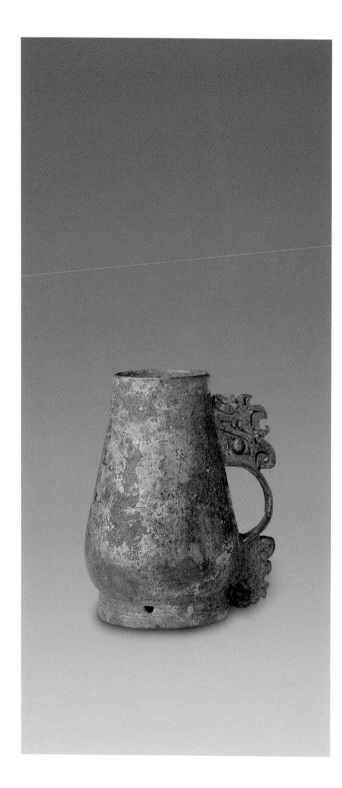

凤首錾觯

西周中期

青铜质

宽 11.9 厘米，通高 14.9 厘米，重 0.72 千克

Zhi with a Phoenix Head Handle

Mid Western Zhou Dynasty

Bronze

Width 11.9 cm/ Height 14.9 cm/ Weight 0.72 kg

敛口，圈足，深腹下垂。一侧半环錾，錾上端饰透雕凤鸟首，錾下方为凤尾状垂珥。1964 年国家文物局调拨。

故宫博物院藏

There is a convergent mouth, a ring foot, and a deep drooping belly. There is a semi-ring handle, the upper of which is decorated with a phoenix-head sculpture and the lower of which with a dropping decoration in the shape of a phoenix-tail. The vessel was allocated from State Administration of Cultural Heritage in 1964.

Preserved in The Palace Museum

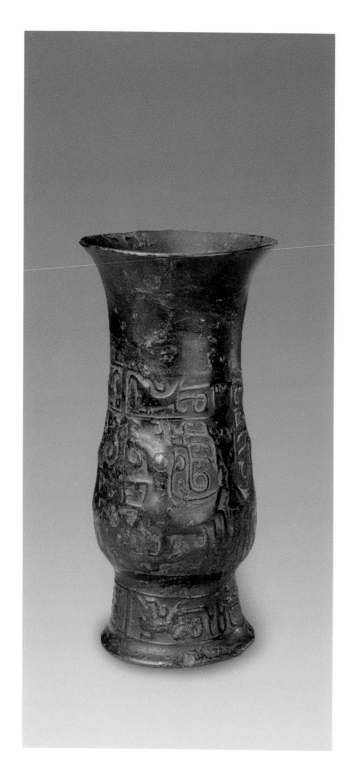

鸟纹觯

西周中期

青铜质

口径 8.3 厘米，通高 14.5 厘米，重 0.38 千克

Zhi with Bird Pattern

Mid Western Zhou Dynasty

Bronze

Mouth Diameter 8.3 cm/ Height 14.5 cm/

Wight 0.38 kg

侈口，颈弧度小，深腹，圈足。饰三道凤鸟纹。清宫旧藏。

故宫博物院藏

The vessel has a wide flared mouth, a neck with a small radian, a deep belly, and a ring foot. The body is decorated with three belts of phoenix patterns. The vessel was originally an antique from the imperial palace of the Qing Dynasty. Preserved in The Palace Museum

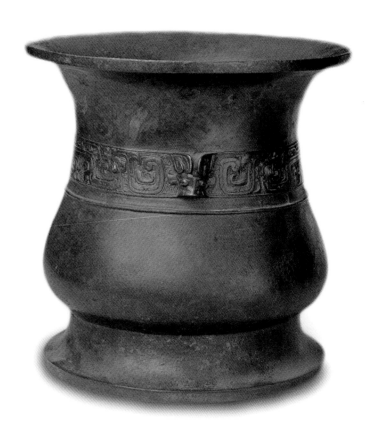

免尊

西周中期

青铜质

宽 18.3 厘米，通高 17.2 厘米，重 2.62 千克

Zun with Character "Mian"

Mid western Zhou Dynasty

Bronze

Width 18.3 cm/ Height 17.2 cm/ Weight 2.62 kg

侈口，圆垂腹，圈足。颈部前后雕铸兽首，兽首两侧均饰垂冠回首的夔鸟纹。尊内底有铭文 5 行 49 字。清宫旧物（原藏颐和园）。

故宫博物院藏

The vessel has a flared mouth, a round and dropping belly, and a ring foot. The anterior and posterior parts of the neck are both decorated with beast head patterns, with Kui dragon and pattern designs on both sides of the heads. There is an inscription of 49 characters in 5 lines on the bottom of the vessel. The vessel was an antique from the imperial palace of the Qing Dynasty (originally kept in the Summer Palace).

Preserved in The Palace Museum

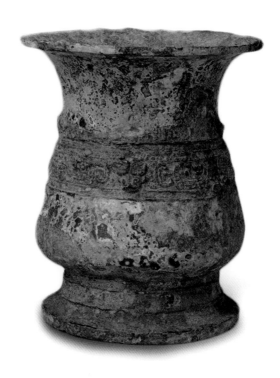

次尊

西周中期

青铜质

宽 16.9 厘米，通高 19.4 厘米，重 1.9 千克

Zun with Character "Ci"

Mid western Zhou Dynasty

Bronze

Width 16.9 cm/ Height 19.4 cm/ Weight 1.9 kg

圆形，侈口，长颈，腹部向下倾垂，圈足。颈部前后有对称的浮雕兽首，兽首两侧饰鸟纹，圈足饰两道弦纹。尊内底铸铭文4行30字。1952年国家文物局调拨。

故宫博物院藏

The vessel has a round body, a large mouth, a long neck, a drooping belly, and a ring foot. The anterior and posterior parts of the neck are both decorated with symmetrical embossed designs of beast head, both sides of which are decorated with bird pattern. The ring foot is decorate with two bands of string patterns There is an inscription of 30 characters in 4 lines on the bottom of the vessel. It was allocated from State Administration of Cultural Heritage in 1952. Preserved in The Palace Museum

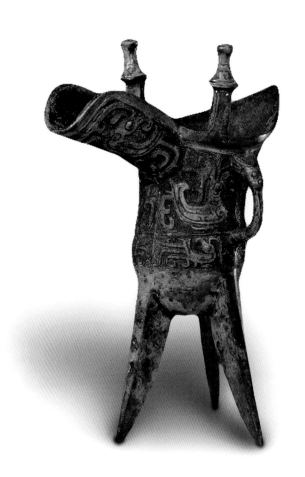

凤鸟纹爵

西周中期

青铜质

口径 17.4 厘米 ×7.5 厘米，通高 22 厘米，重 0.88 千克

Jue with Phoenix and Bird Pattern

Mid Western Zhou Dynasty

Bronze

Calibre 17.4 cm×7.5 cm/ Height 22 cm/ Weight 0.88 kg

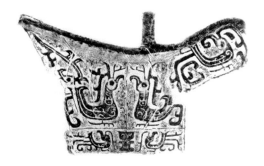

椭圆形，腹较深，圜底，一对帽形柱较高，前有长流，后有尖尾，兽首鋬略小，下具三个刀形尖足。腹及流下饰鸟纹，均以雷纹为地。1946 年入藏。

故宫博物院藏

The oval vessel has a deeper belly, a round bottom, a pair of higher cap-shaped pillar, a long spout before the pillars, and a pointed tail behind the pillars. There is also a smaller beast-head handle and sharp blade-shaped tripodal feet. There are phoenix and bird patterns on the belly and under the spout, with thunder pattern as the ground-tint. It was collected in 1946. Preserved in The Palace Museum

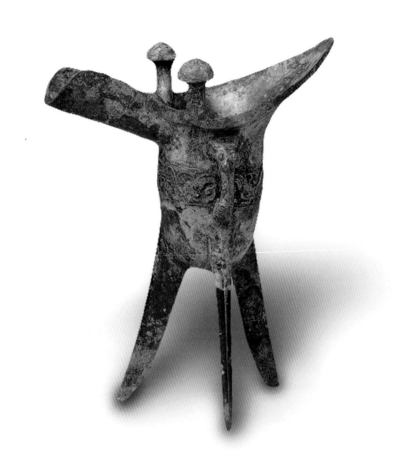

员爵

西周中期

青铜质

宽 16 厘米，通高 18.6 厘米，重 0.66 千克

Jue with Character "Yuan"

Mid Western Zhou Dynasty

Bronze

Width 16 cm/ Height 18.6 cm/ Weight 0.66 kg

圜底，宽流，菌状柱立于流折与鋬之间。腹
饰分尾长鸟，云雷纹衬地。流侧铭文 3 字，
记此爵为员做的祭祀用爵。1954 年收购。

故宫博物院藏

The vessel has a round bottom, a wide spout,
and a mushroom-shaped pillar standing between
the spout fold and the handle. The belly is
decorated with a reedling with separated tails
with cloud and thunder pattern as the ground-
tint. There is an inscription of 3 characters on
the sides of the spout, recording that the vessel
was made by Yuan for use as a sacrificed vessel.
It was acquired in 1954.

Preserved in The Palace Museum

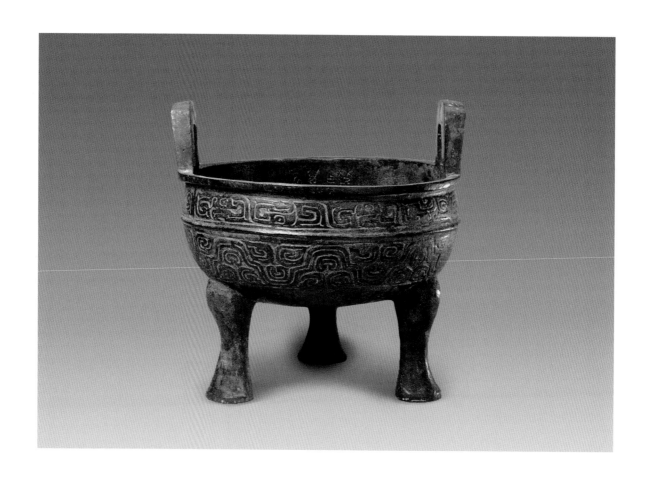

虢文公子㪮鼎

西周晚期

青铜质

宽 30.9 厘米，通高 30 厘米，重 9.08 千克

Tripod with Characters Including "㪮"

Late Western Zhou Dynasty

Bronze

Width 30.9 cm/ Height 30 cm/ Weight 9.08 kg

浅腹，三蹄足，平沿，二直耳。口下饰窃曲纹，腹中部有一道凸弦纹，将下腹部的环带纹与口下窃曲纹带隔开。耳外侧饰重环纹。鼎内侧有铭文4行21字。清宫旧物（原藏颐和园）。

故宫博物院藏

The tripod has a shallow belly, three hoof-shaped legs, a flat edge, and two prick ears. Under the rim of the mouth on the outside, there is ragged curve and there is a streak of protruded string pattern in the middle of the belly, which separates the line-curving wave pattern below the rim of the mouth and a band of wave pattern that surrounds the lower part of the belly. The outside of the ear is decorated with thick ring pattern. In the inner wall of the tripod, there is a 21-character inscription in 4 lines. The tripod belongs to the collection of the imperial palace of the Qing Dynasty (originally collected by the Summer Palace).

Preserved in The Palace Museum

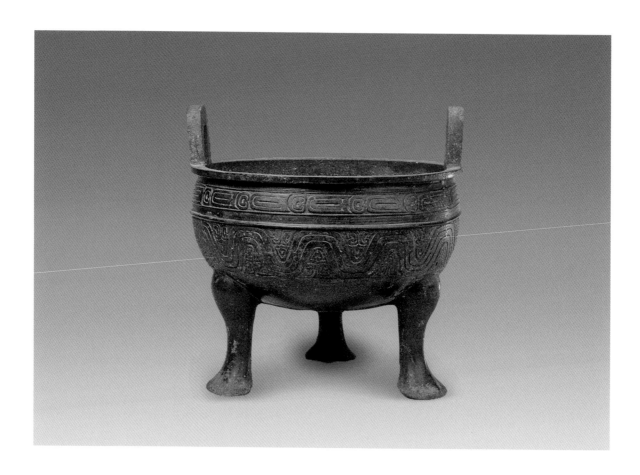

姬嬲鼎

西周晚期

青铜质

宽 28.4 厘米，通高 27.3 厘米，重 6.4 千克

Tripod with Characters "Ji Shang"

Late Western Zhou Dynasty

Bronze

Width 28.4 cm/ Height 27.3 cm/ Weight 6.4 kg

圜底，立耳，蹄足，平沿外折。口下饰重环纹，腹部饰环带纹。内壁铭文 27 字。溥仪留存天津静园文物（后收归故宫）。

故宫博物院藏

The tripod has a round bottom, prick ears, hoof-shaped legs, and a flat edge which is folded outward. The area under the rim of the mouth on the outside is decorated with thick ring patterns and the belly is decorated with big wave pattern that surrounds it. There is an inscription of 27 characters on the inner wall of the tripod. It is a cultural relic left by Pu Yi, the last emperor of the Qing Dynasty, in Jing Yuan (Garden of Serenity) in Tianjin, a place where Pu Yi lived.

Preserved in The Palace Museum

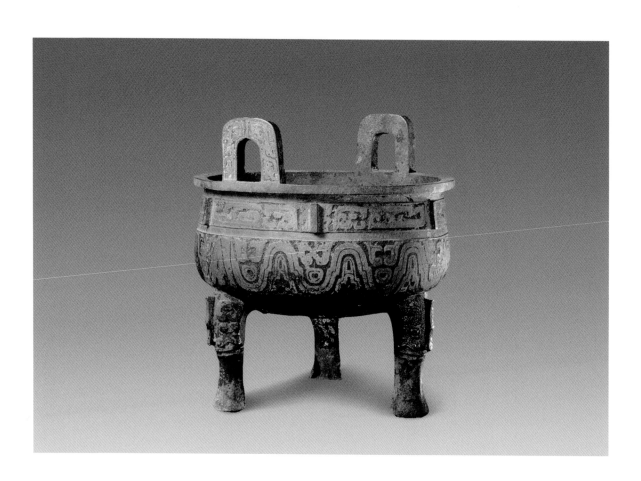

小克鼎

西周晚期

青铜质

宽 33.6 厘米，通高 35.4 厘米，重 12.54 千克

Tripod with Character " Xiao Ke "

Late Western Zhou Dynasty

Bronze

Width 33.6 cm/ Height 35.4 cm/ Weight 12.54 kg

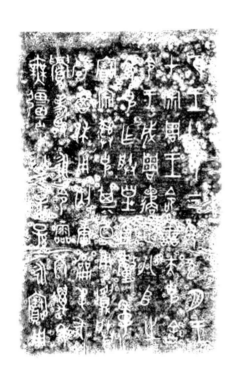

口部微敛，腹略鼓，腹壁厚实，方唇宽沿，立耳，蹄足，形制厚重。颈部饰有三组变形兽面纹，间隔以六道棱脊，腹部饰宽大的环带纹，立耳两侧饰有相对的龙纹，三足上部是突出的兽首。此鼎整体气魄雄浑，威严沉重，纹饰疏朗畅达，不以细致见工。小克鼎内壁铸铭文 8 行 72 字。1956 年冯公度先生捐献。

故宫博物院藏

The tripod has a slightly small mouth, a slightly bulged belly with thick and solid walls, a square lip with a wide edge, two prick ears, and three hoof-shaped legs. The design and modeling of the trip display a sense of dignity and massiveness. On the neck of the tripod, there are three groups of transformed animal-mask designs separated by six vertical ridges. The belly is decorated with a wide band pattern that surrounds it, and both sides of the prick ears are decorated with dragon pattern symmetrical to each other. The upper region of the legs is decorated with protruded animal head. With smooth and succinct pattern rather than exquisite decoration, this tripod is of great forcefulness and powerful stateliness. On its inner wall, there is a 72-character inscription in 8 lines. This tripod was donated by Mr. Feng Gongdu in 1956.

Preserved in The Palace Museum

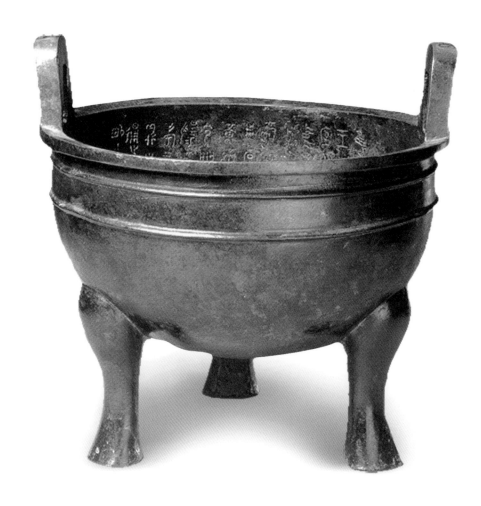

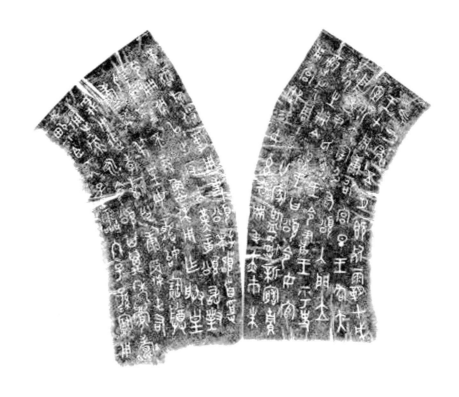

颂鼎

西周晚期

青铜质

宽 30.3 厘米，通高 38.4 厘米，重 7.24 千克

圆腹，圜底，二立耳，腹饰二道弦纹。鼎内壁有铭文 14 行 152 字。清宫旧物（原藏颐和园）。

故宫博物院藏

Tripod with Character "Song"

Late Western Zhou Dynasty

Bronze

Width 30.3 cm/ Height 38.4 cm/ Weight 7.24 kg

The tripod has a round belly, a round bottom, two prick ears, and two streaks of string pattern that decorate the belly. On the inner wall of the tripod, there is an inscription of 152 characters in 14 lines. The tripod is an antique from the collection of the imperial palace of the Qing Dynasty (originally collected in the Summer Palace).

Preserved in The Palace Museum

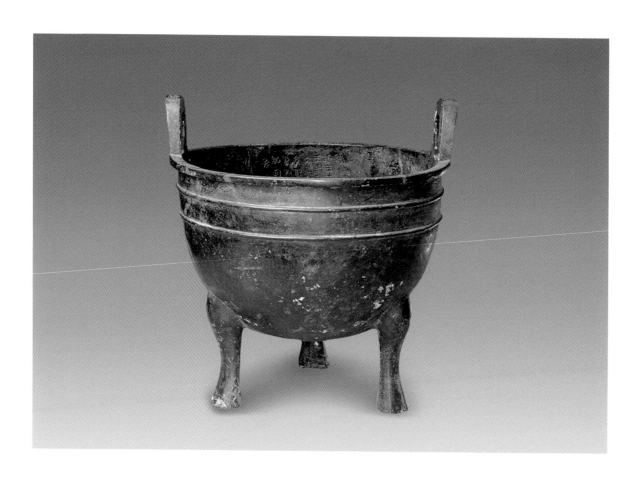

大鼎

西周晚期

青铜质

宽 38.7 厘米，通高 39.7 厘米，重 12.56 千克

Tripod with Character "Da"

Late Western Zhou Dynasty

Bronze

Width 38.7 cm/ Height 39.7 cm/ Weight 12.56 kg

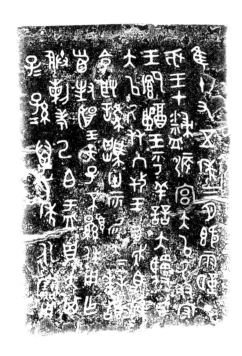

深圆腹，平沿外折，二立耳，三蹄足。口下饰二道弦纹。鼎内有铭文 8 行 82 字。1995 年从上海收购。

故宫博物院藏

The tripod has a deep round belly, a flat edge which is folded outward, two prick ears, and three hoof-shaped feet. Two streaks of string pattern are decorated under the edge. Inside the tripod, there is an 8-line inscription of 82 words. The tripod was acquired in Shanghai in 1995. Preserved in The Palace Museum

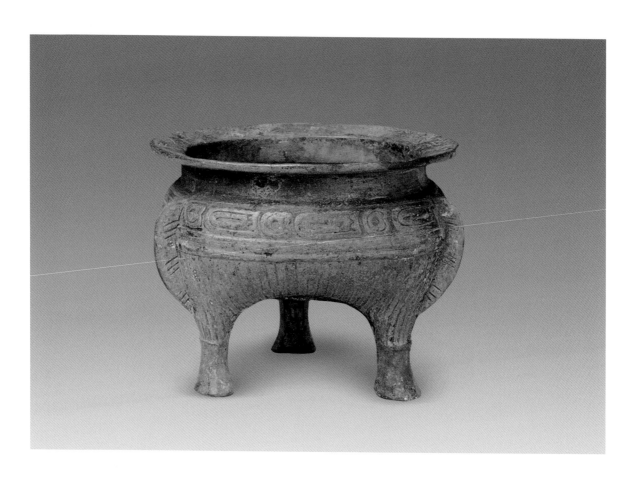

杜伯鬲

西周晚期

青铜质

宽 17.5 厘米，通高 13.2 厘米，重 1.58 千克

Li with Characters "Du Bo"

Late Western Zhou Dynasty

Bronze

Width 17.5 cm/ Height 13.2 cm/ Weight 1.58 kg

宽平缘外折，束颈，圆肩，底部近平，足呈兽蹄形，器身三面出戟。肩部饰重环纹，下腹饰细直纹。铭文 17 字铸在口上。

故宫博物院藏

This cooking vessel has a wide and a flat edge which is folded outward, a narrowed neck, a round shoulder, an almost flat bottom, three hoof-like legs, and three halberds decorating the three sides of the body. Multiple layers of ring patterns are designed on the shoulder, and thin straight pattern is engraved on the lower part of the belly. There is an inscription of 17 words on the edge of the mouth.

Preserved in The Palace Museum

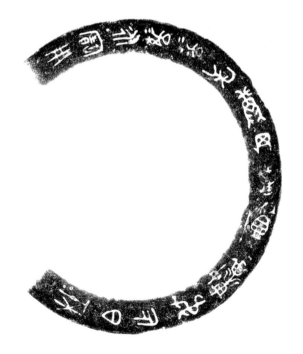

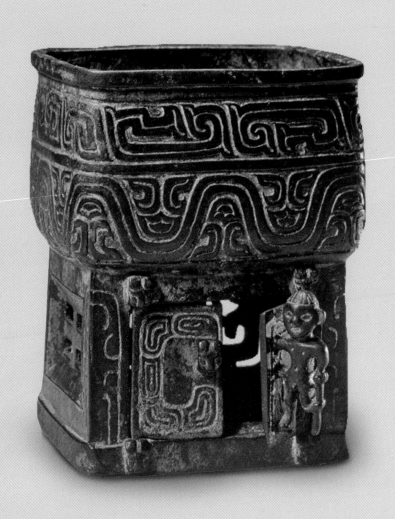

刖人鬲

西周晚期

青铜质

口径 11.2 厘米×9 厘米，通高 13.5 厘米，重 1.46 千克

口沿下饰窃曲纹，腹饰环带纹。平底方座，正面开门，守门者是一个受过刖刑的人的形象，门枢齐全，可以启闭；方座两侧有窗，周饰云纹。背面饰镂空窃曲纹。方座内可燃木炭以温鼎内食物。1959 年北京市文化局调拨（原由倪玉书收藏）。

故宫博物院藏

Li with a Yue Ren Figure

Late Western Zhou Dynasty

Bronze

Mouth Diameter 11.2 cm × 9 cm/ Height 13.5 cm/ Weight 1.46 kg

The vessel is decorated with ragged curve design under its mouth. There is a design of ring patterns on the belly. The body is divided into flat bottom and square pedestal. The pedestal can be opened from the front, and a figure of Yue Ren was cast to stay at the opening as a doorkeeper (Yue Ren refers to a man who was punished by cutting a foot or feet; cutting a man's foot or feet was a cruel punishment in the past in China). There are hinges, and the door can be opened and closed. Two sides of the square pedestal have windows with cloud-like patterns. The back is decorated with hollowed-out waves designs (a kind of flat successive ragged curve). Charcoal can be burned in the pedestal to warm food in the cauldron. The vessel was allocated from Beijing Municipal Bureau of Culture in 1959 and originally collected by Ni Yushu.

Preserved in The Palace Museum

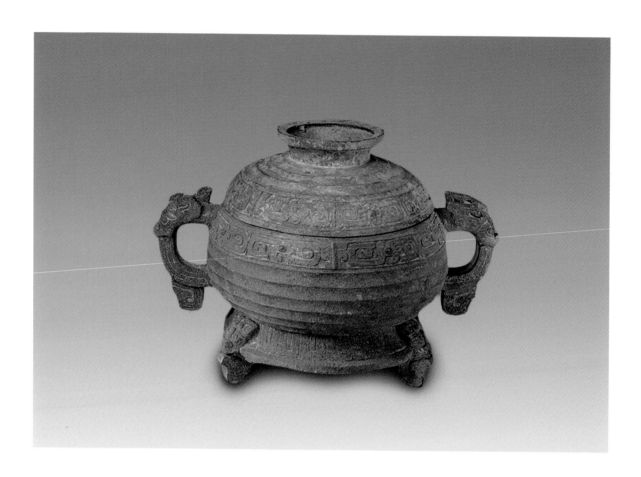

仲枏父簋

西周晚期

青铜质

宽 38.8 厘米，通高 25.5 厘米，重 7.66 千克

Gui with Characters "Zhong Nan Fu"

Late Western Zhou Dynasty

Bronze

Width 38.8 cm/ Height 25.5 cm/ Weight 7.66 kg

圆鼓腹，二兽耳，弇口，圈足下有三短兽首足。有盖，盖顶为圆形捉手。盖面与器腹均饰平行瓦楞文，盖沿及器颈各饰窃曲纹带。簋盖和器上均有铭文 4 行 39 字。1964 年收购。

故宫博物院藏

The vessel has a round swelling belly, a small mouth, a pair of handles in the shape of beasts, and a ring foot with three short feet under it in the shape of a beast head. On the top of the cover there is a round knob handle. Both the upper part of the cover and the belly are decorated with horizontal tile ridge-like patterns. The cover edge and the neck are decorated with a band of the ragged curve. The cover and the body of the vessel are inscribed with 39 characters in 4 lines. It was acquired in 1964.

Preserved in The Palace Museum

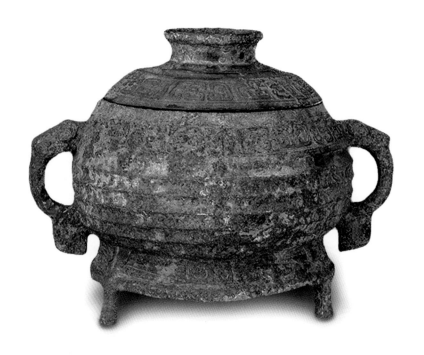

谏簋

西周晚期

青铜质

宽 29.5 厘米，通高 21.2 厘米，重 5.28 千克

Gui with Character "Jian"

Late Western Zhou Dynasty

Bronze

Width 29.5 cm/ Height 21.2 cm/ Weight 5.28 kg

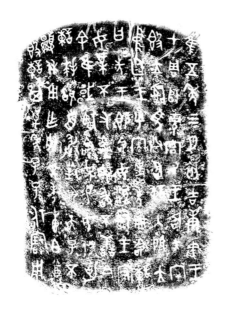

圆形，敛口，鼓腹，圈足下有三小足，腹部两侧兽耳下垂小珥。隆盖，顶有圆形捉手。盖顶和器腹饰瓦纹，器颈与盖沿均饰窃曲纹，圈足饰三角云纹。盖、器对铭，器铭文 9 行 102 字，盖 10 行 101 字。1956 年冯公度先生家属捐献。

故宫博物院藏

This vessel is round in shape with a swelling belly, a convergent mouth, and a ring foot with three short feet under it. On each side of the belly there is a pair of beast-shaped handles with small dropping decoration. On the top of the swelling cover, there is a round knob handle. Both the upper part of the cover and the belly are decorated with tile pattern. The cover edge and the neck of the vessel are decorated with the ragged curve. The ring foot is decorated with cloud pattern. The cover and the body of the vessel are inscribed with 101 characters in 10 lines and 102 characters in 9 lines. It was donated by the family of Mr. Feng Gongdu in 1956.

Preserved in The Palace Museum

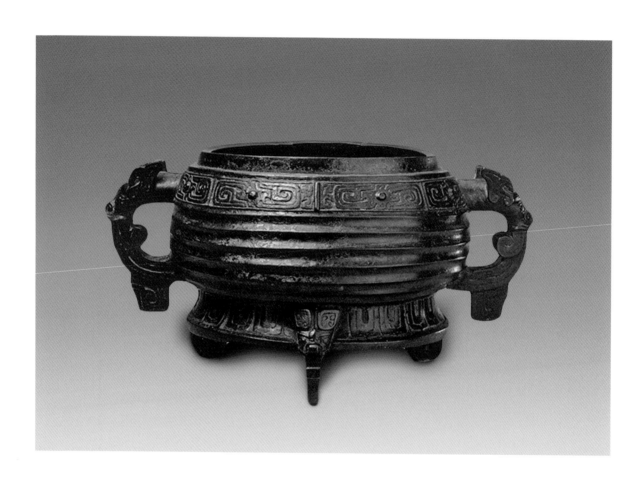

颂簋

西周晚期

青铜质

宽 44.7 厘米，通高 22 厘米，重 10.6 千克

Gui with Character "Song"

Late Western Zhou Dynasty

Bronze

Width 44.7 cm/ Height 22 cm/ Weight 10.6 kg

圆形，敛口，腹部略向下倾垂，二兽耳垂珥。圈足下有卷鼻状小足。颈前、后铸对称的变形兽面，兽面两侧各饰窃曲纹带。腹部饰瓦楞文，圈足饰鳞纹带。簋内底有铭文 15 行 150 字。1956 年冯公度先生家属捐献。

故宫博物院藏

This vessel is round in shape with a convergent mouth, a slightly dropping belly, and a pair of handles in the shape of beasts with a dropping decoration. Under the ring foot there are three small feet in the shape of a curled nose. Both the front and the back part of the neck are symmetrically decorated with the design of transformed beast faces, and on each side of the beast faces there are two bands of ragged curve. The belly is decorated with tile ridge-like patterns, and the ring foot is decorated with a belt of scale-like pattern. There is an inscription of 150 characters in 15 lines on the inner bottom of the vessel. It was donated by the family of Mr. Feng Gongdu in 1956.

Preserved in The Palace Museum

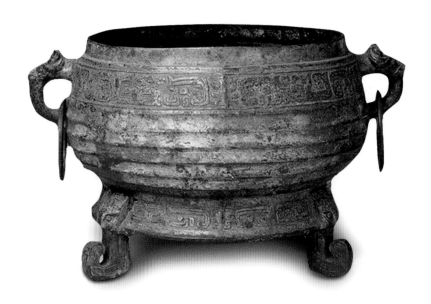

扬簋

西周晚期

青铜质

宽 21.6 厘米，通高 18.7 厘米，重 4 千克

Gui with Character "Yang"

Late Western Zhou Dynasty

Bronze

Width 21.6 cm/ Height 18.7 cm/ Weight 4 kg

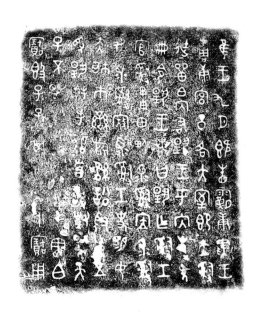

弇口，圆鼓腹。圈足下有三曲折状短足，二附耳各衔套环，器盖已失。器腹饰瓦楞文，颈上与圈足各有一道窃曲纹。圈足上与短足对应处各铸一浮雕兽头。簋内底有铭文 10 行 107 字。1957 年在上海收购。

故宫博物院藏

The vessel has a small mouth, a round and swelling belly. Under the ring foot there are short feet in folded shape. The two looped ears are decorated with loops respectively. The cover is missing. The belly is decorated with tile ridge-like pattern, and both the neck and the ring foot are decorated with ragged curve. On each part of the ring foot that corresponds with the short foot below there is an embossment of beast head. The inner bottom of the vessel is inscribed with 107 characters in 10 lines. It was acquired in Shanghai in 1957.

Preserved in The Palace Museum

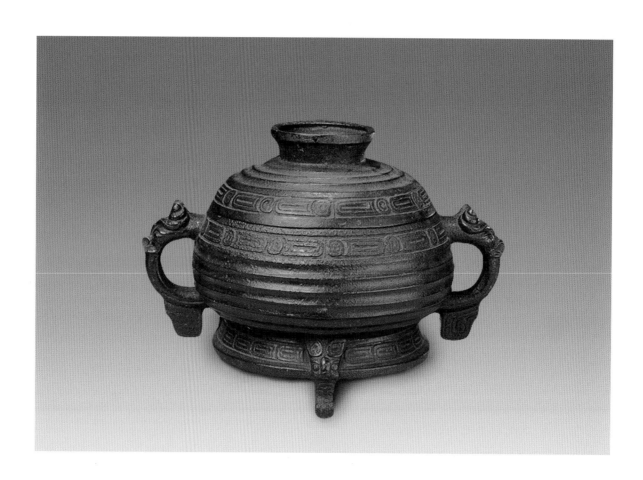

师酉簋

西周晚期

青铜质

宽 32.8 厘米，通高 22.9 厘米，重 4.94 千克

Gui with Characters "Shi You"

Late Western Zhou Dynasty

Bronze

Width 32.8 cm/ Height 22.9 cm/ Weight 4.94 kg

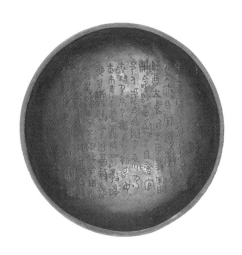

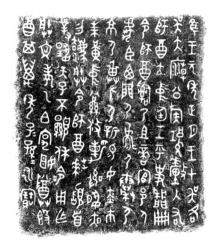

圆形，敛口，鼓腹。有双耳，耳上端雕铸兽头，兽角呈螺旋状。圈足，圈足下有三兽形短足。有盖，盖上有圆形捉手。盖顶与器腹饰瓦纹，盖沿、器颈部和圈足上饰重环纹。盖、器同铭，11 行 106 字。1959 年国家文物局调拨。

故宫博物院藏

This round food vessel has a convergent mouth, a round swelling belly, a pair of handles whose upper parts are cast with a beast head with its horn in spiral shape, and a ring foot under which there are three short feet in the shape of beasts. On the top of the cover there is a round knob handle. The surface of the cover and the belly are decorated with tile pattern. The cover edge, the neck, and the ring foot are decorated with multiple circles pattern. Both the cover and the body are inscribed with the same 106 characters in 11 lines. This vessel was allocated from State Administration of Cultural Heritage in 1959.

Preserved in The Palace Museum

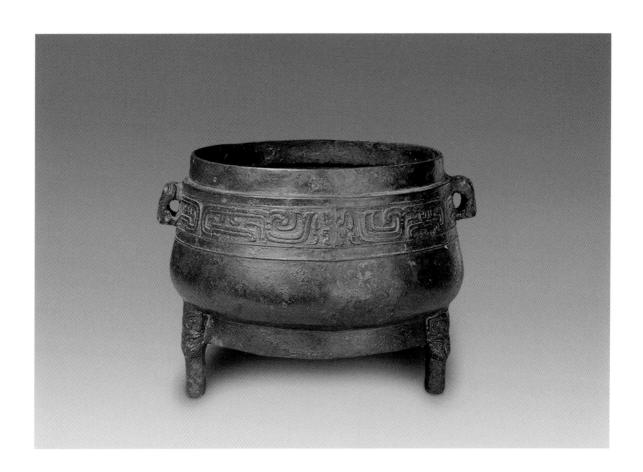

大簋

西周晚期

青铜质

宽 22.2 厘米，通高 14.8 厘米，重 2.7 千克

Gui with Character "Da"

Late Western Zhou Dynasty

Bronze

Width 22.2 cm/ Height 14.8 cm/ Weight 2.7 kg

弇口，鼓腹，兽头衔环耳，环已失，圈足下置三矮附足。颈部饰窃曲纹，前、后正中加饰兽首。圈足与附足对应处有浮雕兽首。内底有铭文 40 字。清宫旧物（原藏颐和园）。

故宫博物院藏

This vessel has a small mouth and a swelling belly. There is a pair of handles in the shape of a beast head with a ring in its mouth (the ring is lost). Below the ring foot there are three short attached feet. The neck is decorated with ragged curve, and on the center of its front and back sides, beast heads are cast. On each area of the ring foot that corresponds with the attached foot below there is decoration with an embossment of a beast head. The inner area of the bottom of the vessel is inscribed with 40 characters. It was an antique of the imperial palace of the Qing Dynasty (originally kept in the Summer Palace). Preserved in The Palace Museum

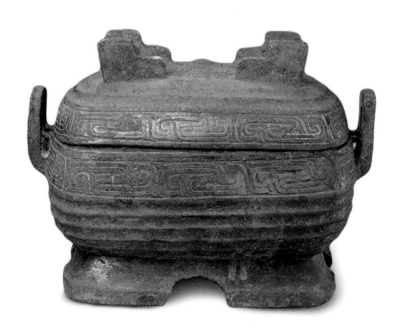

圃盨

西周晚期

青铜质

宽 29.5 厘米，通高 20.4 厘米，重 5.3 千克

Xu with Character "Pu"

Late Western Zhou Dynasty

Bronze

Width 29.5 cm/ Height 20.4 cm/ Weight 5.3 kg

附耳，圈足有缺，盖上有四个矩形足。盖中心饰窃曲纹，盖上与器腹均饰瓦纹，盖沿和颈部各饰窃曲纹带。盖、器同铭，有铭文15字。1957年国家文物局调拨。

故宫博物院藏

This vessel has two looped ears and a misshapen ring foot. There are four rectangular shaped feet on the top of the cover. The center of the cover is decorated with ragged curve. The surface of the cover and the belly are decorated with tile pattern. The cover edge and the neck are respectively decorated with a belt of ragged curve. Both the cover and the belly are inscribed with the same 15 characters. This vessel was allocated from State Administration of Cultural Heritage in 1957.

Preserved in The Palace Museum

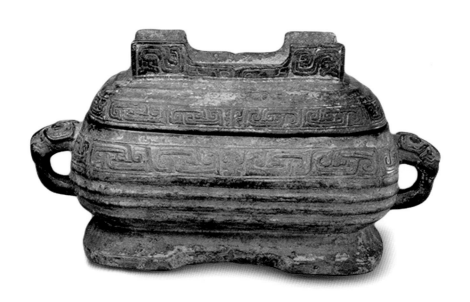

杜伯盨

西周晚期

青铜质

宽 37.3 厘米，通高 36.8 厘米，重 5.66 千克

Xu with Characters "Du Bo"

Late Western Zhou Dynasty

Bronze

Width 37.3 cm/ Height 36.8 cm/ Weight 5.66 kg

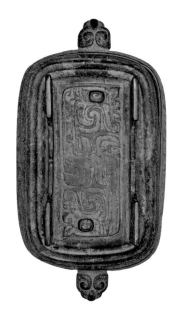

长圆形，敛口，二兽首耳，有盖，盖上有扁足，打开后可以却置。器颈与盖沿各饰窃曲纹带，盖上与器腹均饰瓦楞文。盨盖与器同铭，4 行 30 字。光绪二十年 (1894) 陕西韩城、澄城交界处出土，1946 年入藏。

故宫博物院藏

This vessel has an ovale shape with two handles shaped in a beast head, a convergent mouth, and a cover with flat feet on the top. The cover can serve as another vessel when it is removed from the vessel it covers. The neck and the cover edge are respectively decorated with a belt of ragged curve. The surface of the cover and the belly are decorated with tile-ridge pattern. Both the cover and the belly are inscribed with the same 30 characters in 4 lines. It was unearthed from the border of Hancheng City and Chengcheng County of Shaanxi Province in 1894. It was collected in 1946.

Preserved in The Palace Museum

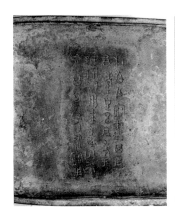

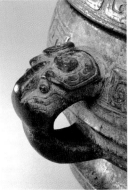

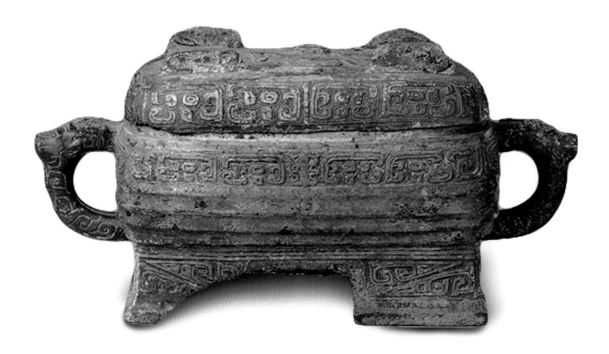

伯孝鼓盨

西周晚期

青铜质

宽 32.8 厘米，通高 15.1 厘米，重 3.67 千克

椭方形，弇口，鼓腹，兽首双耳，圈足外侈，并有缺。盖上有四
扁足，可以却置。盖顶、盖沿与器颈部均饰窃曲纹，腹饰瓦楞纹，
足上饰三角云纹。盖、器同铭，盖 14 字，器 15 字。1957 年收购。

故宫博物院藏

Xu with Characters "Bo Xiao Gu"

Late Western Zhou Dynasty

Bronze

Width 32.8cm/ Height 15.1cm/ Weight 3.67 kg

This oval and square vessel has a small mouth, a swelling belly, a pair
of handles in the shape of a beast head. The ring foot extends outward
with a breach. There are four flat feet on the top of the cover. The cover
can also serve as a vessel when it is removed from the vessel it covers.
The cover top and edge and the neck of the vessel are all decorated
with ragged curve. The belly is decorated with tile pattern, and the
ring foot is decorated with triangular cloud-like pattern. Both the cover
and the belly are inscribed with characters: the cover has 15 characters
inscribed, and the body of the vessel has 14 characters inscribed. It was
collected in 1957.

Preserved in The Palace Museum

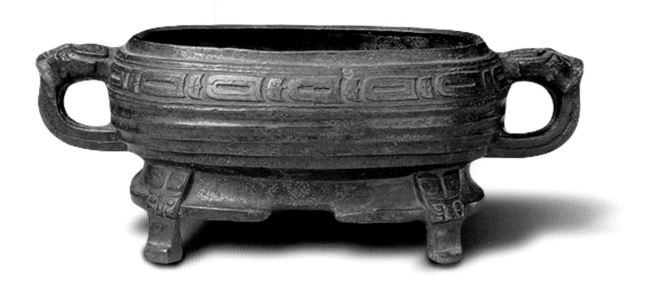

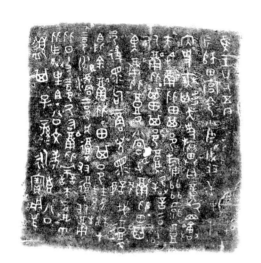

鬲比盨

西周晚期

青铜质

宽 38.9 厘米，通高 14 厘米，重 4.58 千克

器呈长形圆角，敛口，二兽首耳。圈足下有四短足，短足上端雕饰兽头。口下饰重环纹带，腹饰瓦楞文。盨内底有铭文 12 行 139 字。1957 年收购。

故宫博物院藏

Xu with Characters Including " 鬲 "

Late Western Zhou Dynasty

Bronze

Width 38.9 cm/ Height 14 cm/ Weight 4.58 kg

This vessel is long shaped with round corners, and has a convergent mouth, a pair of handles in the shape of a beast head, and a ring foot under which there are four short feet with their upper part decorated with beast head. On the area below the rim of the mouth there is a pattern of multiple circles, and the belly is decorated with tile-ridge pattern. The inner area of the bottom of the container is inscribed with 139 characters in 12 lines. It was acquired in 1957.

Preserved in The Palace Museum

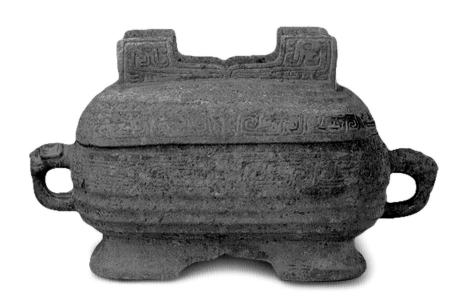

师克盨

西周晚期

青铜质

宽 37.5 厘米，通高 21 厘米，重 5.26 千克

Xu with Characters "Shi Ke"

Late Western Zhou Dynasty

Bronze

Width 37.5 cm/ Height 21 cm/ Weight 5.26 kg

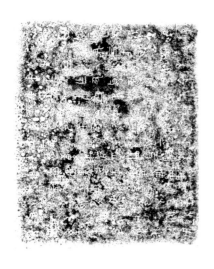

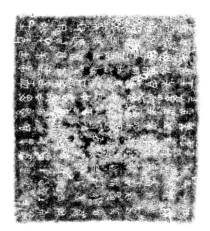

长方形圆角，敛口，圈足，双兽耳，有盖，盖上有四个呈矩形的短足。盖沿与器颈各饰窃曲纹一道。盖上与器腹均饰瓦楞文。盖矩足上饰夔纹。盨盖与器有对铭，14 行 148 字。清光绪年间出土于陕西扶风，1960 年国家文物局调拨。

故宫博物院藏

The vessel is in rectangular shape with rounded corners, a ring foot, two handles shaped like animals, a convergent mouth, and a cover with four short rectangular feet. The cover edge and the neck are decorated with ragged curve, and the cover top and the belly are adorned with title ridge pattern. The rectangular feet of the cover are decorated with Kui dragon design. The inscription of the cover corresponds with that of the body of the vessel. The inscription runs in 148 characters in 14 lines. It was unearthed from Fufeng County, Shaanxi Province, in the years of the reign of Emperor Guangxu of the Qing Dynasty. This vessel was allocated from State Administration of Cultural Heritage in 1960. Preserved in The Palace Museum

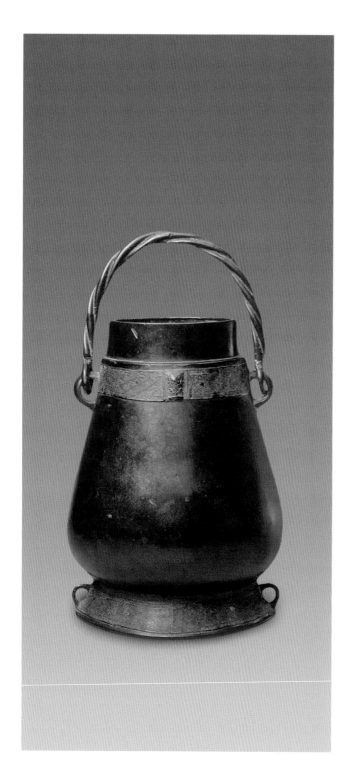

虢季子组卣

西周晚期

青铜质

宽 21.4 厘米，通高 33 厘米，重 5.8 千克

You with Characters "Guo Ji Zi Zu"

Late Shang Dynasty

Bronze

Width 21.4 cm/ Height 33 cm/ Weight 5.8 kg

扁圆形，失盖。器以半环衔接提梁，腹下部
鼓出，圈足两侧铸环钮。器颈与圈足均饰回
纹带，皆夹以联珠纹。器颈在回纹间加饰小
兽首。卣内底有铭文3行17字。1957年收购。

故宫博物院藏

The vessel has a flattened circular shape with its
cover missing. The hoop handle is interlinked
with the vessel by semi-rings. The lower part
of the belly is swelling and there is a ring knob
cast on both the right and left sides of the ring
foot. The neck and the ring foot are decorated
with a belt of fret patterns, mixed with patterns
of a string of beads. Designs of small animal
heads are added among the fret patterns. There
is an inscription of 17 characters in 3 lines on
the inner area of the bottom. The vessel was
acquired in 1957.

Preserved in The Palace Museum

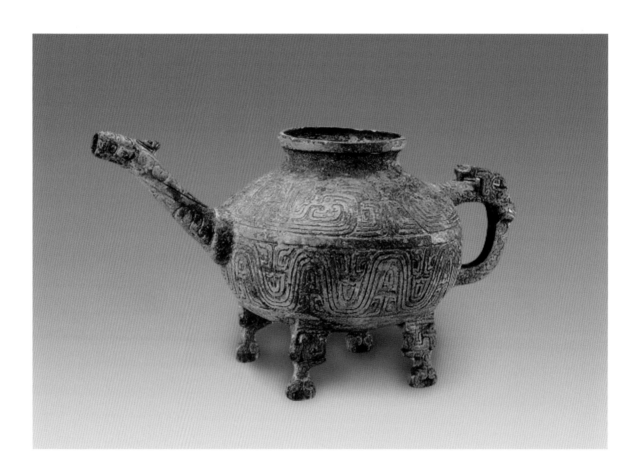

环带纹盉

西周晚期

青铜质

通高 20.5 厘米

He with Girdle Pattern

Late Western Zhou Dynasty

Bronze

Height 20.5 cm

圆口深腹，腹饰环带纹。前有管状流，
后有鋬，与流相对，下承四足。用于盛酒，
调和酒味浓淡。

湖北省博物馆藏

This wine vessel has a round mouth, a
deep belly with girdle pattern, and a spout
on the front, a handle at the back that is
opposite to the spout, and four feet at the
bottom. This served as a vessel to regulate
taste of wine.

Preserved in Hubei Provincial Museum

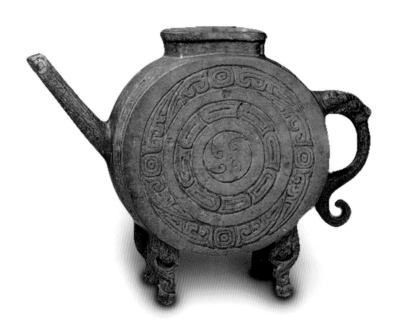

兽錾盉

西周晚期

青铜质

宽 33.8 厘米，通高 24.3 厘米，重 2.92 千克

He with Handle in the Shape of an Animal

Late Western Zhou Dynasty

Bronze

Width 33.8 cm/ Height 24.3 cm/ Weight 2.92 kg

体呈侧置的鼓形，上有圆角方形口，下具四扁足，长管流，盉鋬呈回首龙形。腹饰重环纹、斜角雷纹和圆涡纹，足饰夔龙。这是西周晚期一种特殊的盉。造型别致，独具风格。1964 年入藏。

故宫博物院藏

The vessel body is in the shape of a drum. There is an oval-shaped mouth above and four flattened legs below. There is a long tubular spout. The handle is shaped into a dragon that looks back. There is multiple rings pattern, thunder pattern with oblique angles, and round spiral pattern on the belly, and there is Kui dragon design on the legs, the one in the front stands opposite the one in the back. It is a special wine vessel made in late Western Zhou Dynasty with a unique style. The vessel was collected in 1964.

Preserved in The Palace Museum

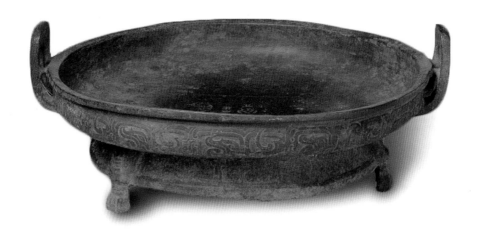

塱汤叔盘

西周晚期

青铜质

宽 40.7 厘米，通高 14.2 厘米，重 6.1 千克

Plate with Characters Including " 塱 "

Late Western Zhou Dynasty

Bronze

Width 40.7 cm/ Height 14.2 cm/ Weight 6.1 kg

平沿方唇，浅腹，两附耳高出器口。圈足低而外撇，下附三兽足。腹部与圈足均饰兽带纹。内底有铭文 29 字。章乃器先生捐献。

故宫博物院藏

The edge of the plate is flat and the lip is square. There is a shallow belly, a pair of ears protruding higher out of the rim of the mouth. The ring leg is short, under which there are three beast feet designs. Both the belly and the ring foot are decorated with belts of beast patterns. There is an inscription of 29 characters on the inner bottom of the place. It was donated by Mr. Zhang Naiqi.

Preserved in The Palace Museum

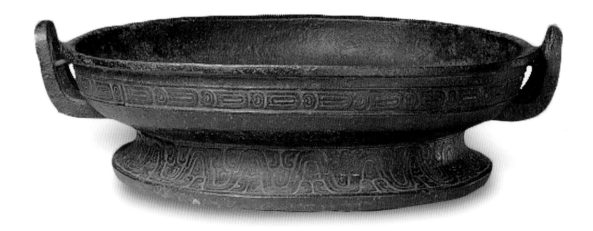

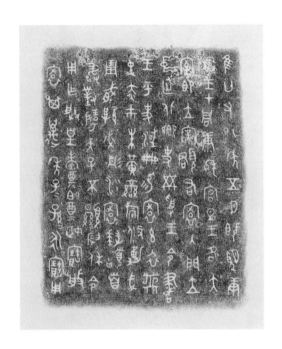

裘盘

西周晚期

青铜质

宽 45.5 厘米，通高 12.9 厘米，重 7.96 千克

圆形，折沿，附耳，圈足。腹饰重环纹，圈足饰环带纹。盘内底铸铭文 10 行 103 字。

1957 年国家文物局调拨。

故宫博物院藏

Plate with Character "裘"

Late Western Zhou Dynasty

Width 45.5 cm/ Height 12.9 cm/ Weight 7.96 kg

The plate is round in shape, with folded edges, a pair of ears on the belly, and a ring foot. The belly is decorated with multiple circles on the belly. The ring foot is decorated with girdle pattern. There is an inscription of 103 characters in 10 lines on the inner bottom. The plate was allocated from State Administration of Cultural Heritage in 1957.

Preserved in The Palace Museum

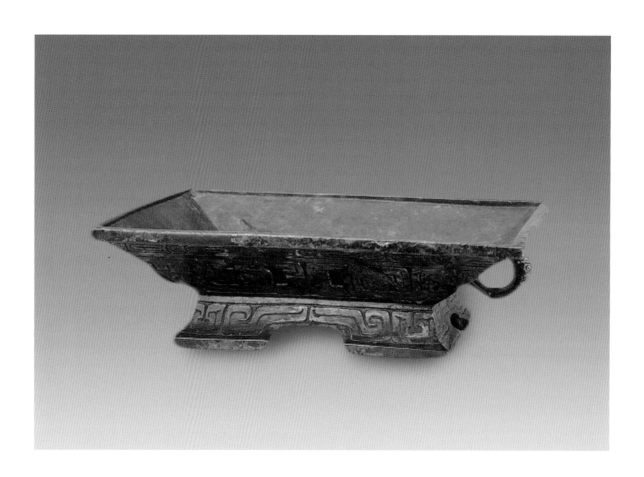

芮太子白簠

西周晚期

青铜质

宽 33.9 厘米，通高 8.9 厘米，重 5.36 千克

Fu with Characters "Rui Tai Zi Bai"

Late Western Zhou Dynasty

Bronze

Width 33.9 cm/ Height 8.9 cm/ Weight 5.36 kg

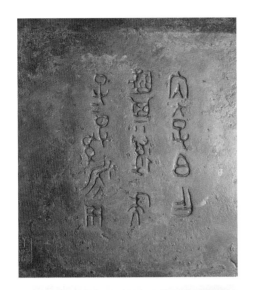

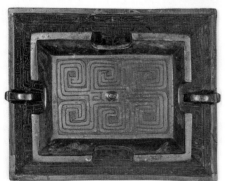

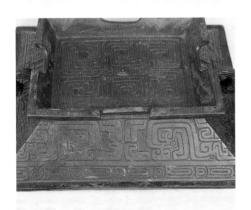

腹壁斜收，方圈足前后正中有缺，腹左右两侧有环耳，耳上端雕饰兽头。腹饰兽带纹，足饰窃曲纹，口沿饰重环纹。内底铭文 3 行 14 字。1957 年国家文物局调拨。

故宫博物院藏

The belly of the vessel is oblique inward. There is a notch designed on the forepart and the back of the ring foot. Laterally on the belly, there are two ring ears, on the top of which beast-head pattern is sculptured. The belly is decorated with belts of beast-like pattern. The foot is decorated with impoverished curves. The rim of the mouth is decorated with Qie Qu designs. There is an inscription of 14 characters in 3 lines on the inner bottom. It was allocated from State Administration of Cultural Heritage in 1957. Preserved in The Palace Museum

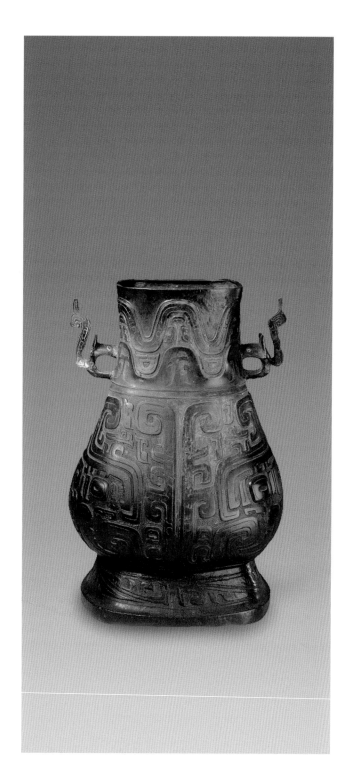

兽面纹壶

西周晚期

青铜质

宽 33 厘米，通高 48.2 厘米，重 14.64 千克。

Bronze Pot with Animal Mask Pattern

Late Western Zhou Dynasty

Bronze

Width 33 cm/ Height 48.2 cm/ Weight 14.64 kg

形体高大，呈椭圆形，宽颈，深腹，圈足。壶颈部饰两对长尾高冠回首的凤鸟纹，十分华丽。颈两侧有三象头为耳，象鼻高高翘起，形象生动逼真，每个象耳内各套铸一绳纹大环。器腹饰兽面纹，以细云雷纹为地。口下与圈足均饰连续的环带纹，环带内又施口眉图案。清宫旧藏。

故宫博物院藏

The large and tall pot has an oval-shaped body, a broad neck, a deep belly and a ring foot. The neck of the vessel is decorated with two couples of phenix patterns with long tails and high-standing crowns, which are gorgeous in appearance. The ears on both sides of the neck of the vessel are in the shape of a vivid elephant head, with noses turning up. Each pattern of the elephant ear has a cord mark. The belly of the vessel is decorated with a design of beast face, with delicate clouds and thunder design as ground-tint. The lower-section of the mouth and the ring foot are both decorated with successive girdle-shaped patterns, with a mouth and eyebrow pattern inside the girdle-shaped pattern. The utensil was an an tique from the imperial palace of the Qing Danasty.

Preserved in The Palace Museum

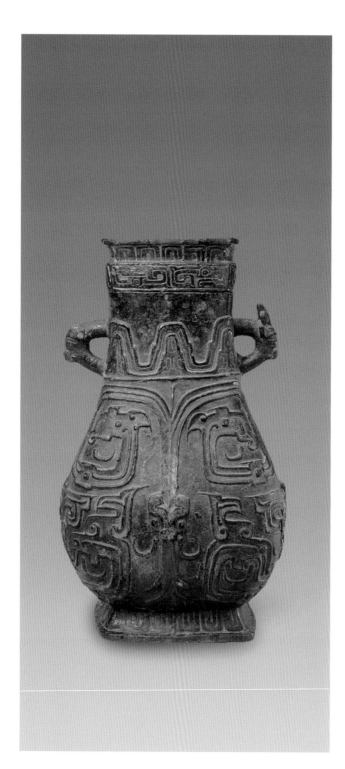

芮公壶

西周晚期

青铜质

宽 22 厘米，通高 37.6 厘米，重 9.45 千克

Bronze Pot with Characters "Rui Gong"

Late Western Zhou Dynasty

Bronze

Width 22 cm/ Height 37.6 cm/ Weight 9.45 kg

椭圆形器体，平顶盖，有圈形捉手。器身直口，长颈，深腹稍鼓，兽首形耳，圈足。捉手与圈足饰鳞纹，盖沿饰窃曲纹，器颈饰环带纹。器腹饰双尾龙纹，以龙首为中心，体躯向两侧展开。盖上铸铭文9字。记芮公铸造随行用壶，永宝用它。清宫旧藏。

故宫博物院藏

The pot has an oval-shaped body and a cover with a flattened top with ring handles. The vessel has a straight mouth, a long neck, and a deep belly with a relatively swelling shape. The ears are in the shape of beast head. There is a ring foot for this vessel. The handles and ring foot are both decorated with scale pattern; the rim of the cover is decorated with Qie Qu pattern; the neck of the vessel is decorated with girdle-like pattern. The belly is decorated with a double-tail dragon pattern, with the dragon head in the middle and the body stretching to the direction of two flanks. There is an inscription of 9 characters on the surface of the cover. The content of the inscription is about Rui Gong making this pot as water bottle and treating it as a permanent treasure. It was originally a collection in the imperial palace of the Qing Dynasty. Preserved in The Palace Museum

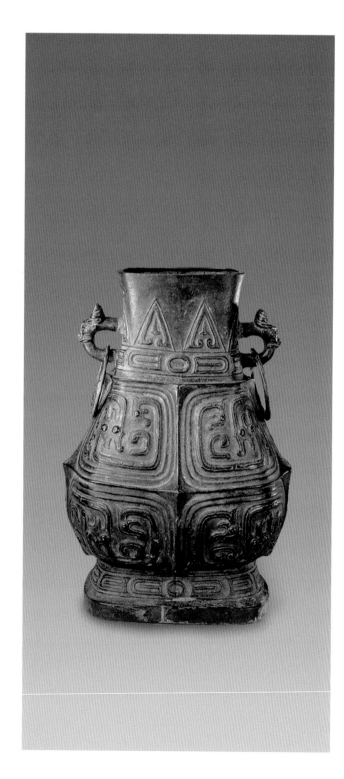

蔡公子壶

西周晚期

青铜质

宽 29.6 厘米，通高 40.2 厘米，重 9.22 千克

Pot with Characters "Cai Gong Zi"

Late Western Zhou Dynasty

Bronze

Width 29.6 cm/ Height 40.2 cm/ Weight 9.22 kg

直口，长颈，兽首形大套环双耳，鼓腹，圈足有宽边。壶盖已失。壶口下饰三角形兽面纹，器颈及圈足饰重环纹，器腹两面以突起带纹构成田字形网格。其间每一空格均饰蟠龙纹。壶底铸铭文7 行 29 字。1956 年冯公度先生家属捐献。

故宫博物院藏

The cover of the utensil is lost. The pot has a straight mouth, a long neck, two ears in the shape of a beast head equipped with a big hitched ring, a swelling belly, and a ring foot with broad margin. The lower-section of the mouth of the utensil is decorated with design of beast face in the shape of a triangle. The neck and the ring foot are both decorated with multiple rings pattern. The anterior and posterior sides of the utensil belly are decorated with convex grid-like patterns bearing resemblance to the Chinese character " 田 ". Each smaller box of the grid is decorated with curled-up dragon pattern. There is an inscription of 29 characters in 7 lines on the bottom. This relic was donated by the family of Mr. Feng Gongdu in 1956.

Preserved in The Palace Museum

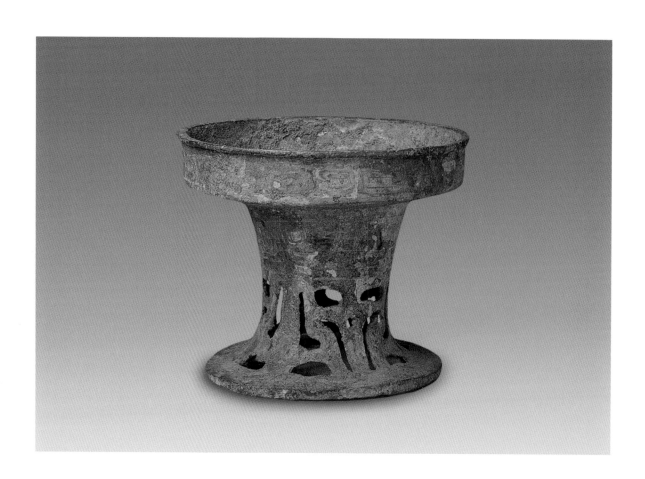

重环纹豆

西周晚期

青铜质

宽 23 厘米，通高 20.8 厘米，重 2.5 千克

Dou with Multiple Rings Pattern

Late Western Zhou Dynasty

Bronze

Width 23 cm/ Height 20.8 cm/ Weight 2.5 kg

浅盘，直口，束腰，高足。盘沿饰重环纹，圈足饰透雕兽带纹。1964 年入藏。

故宫博物院藏

The vessel has a shallow pan, with a straight mouth, a slender waist, and a tall ring foot. The edge of the pan is decorated with a multiple rings pattern, and the ring foot is decorated with deep carved belt of beast pattern. The vessel was collected in 1964.

Preserved in The Palace Museum

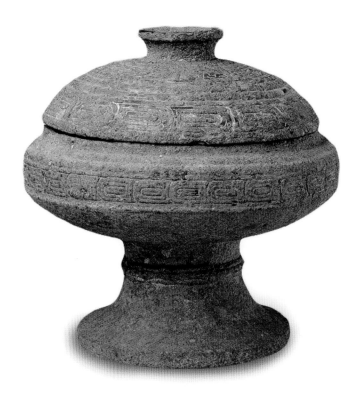

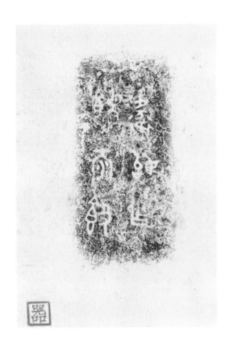

卫始豆

西周晚期

青铜质

宽 18.5 厘米，通高 17.4 厘米，重 2.3 千克

敛口，圈底，浅盘，高足，隆盖圈握。盖顶饰瓦纹，盖沿与器上均饰重环纹，足饰粗弦纹一周。盖与器同铭，均 2 行 6 字，记卫始自做灵簋。

故宫博物院藏

Dou With Character "Wei Shi"

Late Zhou Dynasty

Bronze

Width 18.5 cm/ Height 17.4 cm/ Weight 2.3 kg

The vessel has a convergent mouth, a round bottom, a round bottom, a shallow plate, and a high foot. It also has a raised cover with a knob for hand holding. The outer surface of the cover is decorated with tile pattern, and the rim along the mouth and the body of the vessel are decorated with multiple circles pattern, the foot with a circle of thick bowstring pattern. The inscriptions on the cover and the body of the vessel are the same, all having 6 characters in 2 lines, recording that Wei Shi made this vessel.

Preserved in The Palace Museum

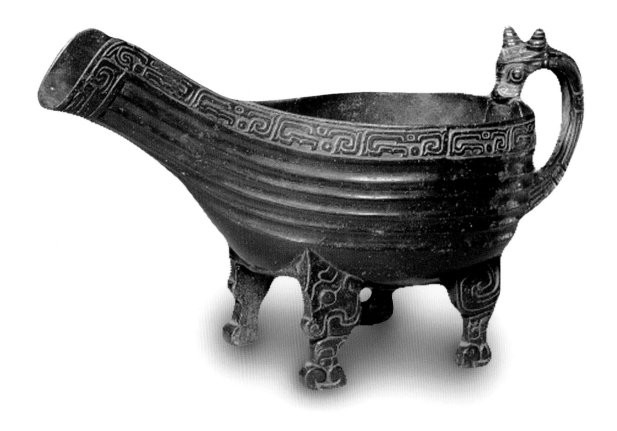

郳□子商匜

西周晚期

青铜质

长 42.3 厘米，通高 22.1 厘米，重 2.1 千克

曲口，直唇，前有宽流，后设兽首鋬。腹饰瓦楞纹，口下饰窃曲纹。内底有铭文 16 字。1958 年收购。

故宫博物院藏

Yi with Characters "Ju □ Zi Shang"

Late Western Zhou Dynasty

Length 42.3 cm/ Height 22.1 cm/ Weight 2.1 kg

The mouth is crooked and the lips are straight. On the front part of the vessel, there is wide spout, and on the back there is a handle with designs of animal head. The belly of this vessel is decorated with tile ridges, and the rim of the mouth with ragged curve. There is an inscription of 16 characters on the inner side of the bottom. It was acquired in 1958.

Preserved in The Palace Museum

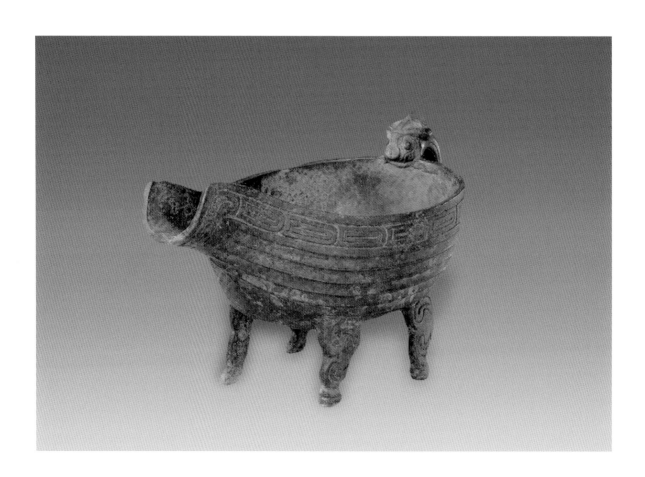

叔男父匜

西周晚期

青铜质

长 26.2 厘米，通高 15.3 厘米，重 1.92 千克

Yi with Characters "Shu Nan Fu"

Late Western Zhou Dynasty

Bronze

Length 26.2 cm/ Height 15.3 cm/ Weight 1.92 kg

口缘较直，流槽窄长，深腹，圜底，四条扁
兽足，后部有龙形鋬。内底有铭文 22 字，
记叔男父为其女儿霍姬做陪嫁用匜。1960 年
收购。

故宫博物院藏

The bronze artifact has a long narrow spout and
a straight mouth. It has a deep belly and a round
bottom supported with four flat animal legs
designs. The handle is in the shape of a dragon.
There is an inscription of 22 characters on the
inner side of the bottom of the vessel, recording
that the man sent this bronze to his daughter
named Huo Ji as her dowry. It was acquired in
1960.

Preserved in The Palace Museum

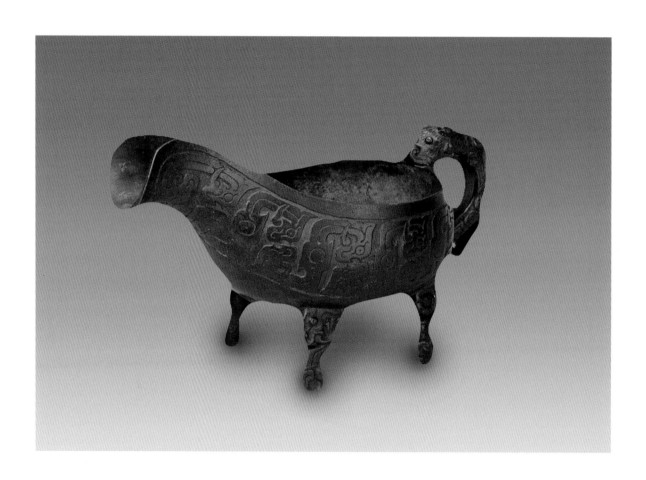

叔上匜

西周晚期

青铜质

长 28.6 厘米，通高 16.8 厘米，重 1.86 千克

Yi with Characters "Shu Shang"

Late Western Zhou Dynasty

Bronze

Length 28.6 cm/ Height 16.8 cm/ Weight 1.86 kg

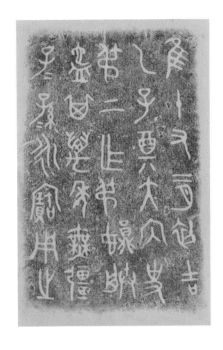

宽流，曲口。錾呈夔龙状，口衔匜沿，呈探水状。器腹饰兽带纹。匜的前两足上部饰兽首，后两足上部为兽尾。内底有铭文 5 行 33 字。

故宫博物院藏

The bronze artifact has a wide spout and a bent mouth. The handle is designed in the shape of a Kui dragon whose mouth takes "Yi" rim to pose to stretch out for water. The belly is decorated with animal band patterns. The upper part of the two front legs is decorated with animal heads, while the two back legs with animal tails. There is an inscription of 33 characters in 5 lines.
Preserved in The Palace Museum

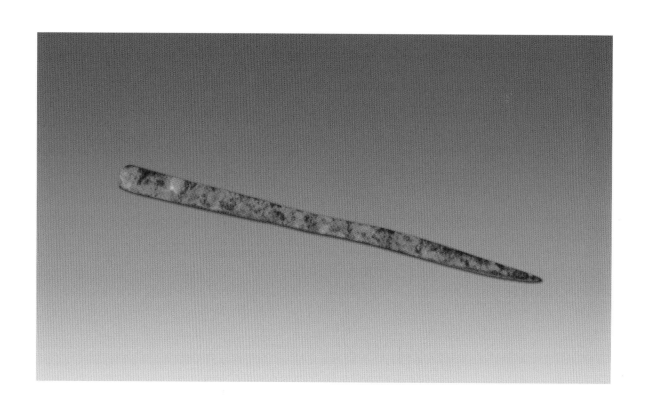

青铜针

西周

青铜质

通长 9.2 厘米

针体呈三棱形，末端尖锐。可以用于放血、刺病。

陕西扶风县齐家村出土。

宝鸡市周原博物馆藏

Bronze Needle

Western Zhou Dynasty

Bronze

Length 9.2 cm

It is a triple-prism-shaped needle with a sharp end used for bloodletting and puncture treatment. It was unearthed in Qijia Village, Fufeng County, Shaanxi Province.

Preserved in Zhouyuan Museum, Baoji City

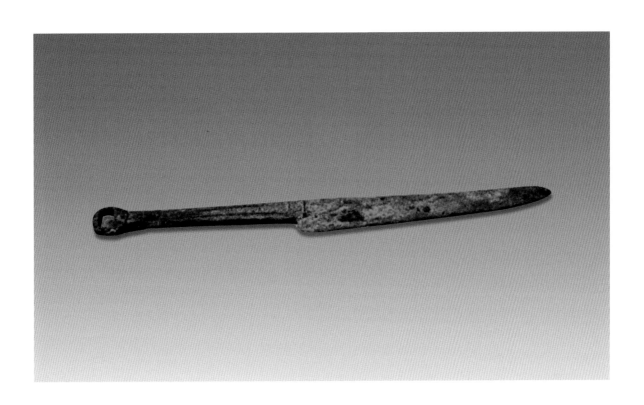

青铜刀

西周

青铜质

通长 21.3 厘米

柄：长 5.5 厘米

刃：宽 2.5 厘米

西周人生活中使用的刀具，亦可用于体表手术。

1983 年陕西扶风县齐家村采集。

宝鸡市周原博物馆藏

Bronze Knife

Western Zhou Dynasty

Bronze

Length 21.3 cm

Handle: Length 5.5 cm

Blade: Width 2.5 cm

This knife was used in the daily life of the people in Western Zhou Dynasty and for body surface surgery as well. It was collected from Qijia Village, Fufeng County, Shaanxi Province, in 1983.

Preserved in Zhouyuan Museum, Baoji City

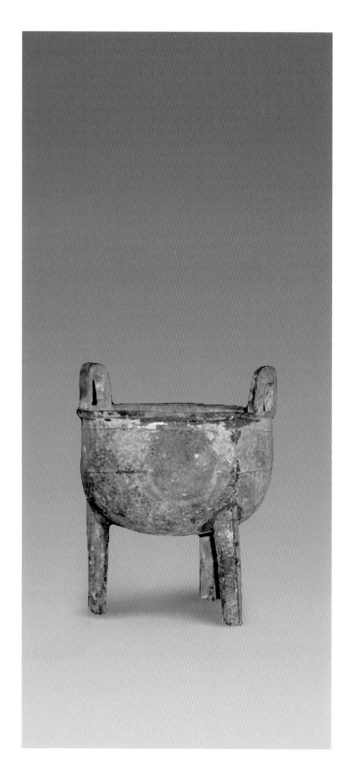

铜鼎

西周

青铜质

口径 15.5 厘米，底径 12 厘米，通高 19 厘米，

重 1.7 千克

Bronze Tripod

Western Zhou Dynasty

Bronze

Mouth Diameter 15.5 cm/ Bottom Diameter

12 cm/ Height 19 cm/ Weight 1.7 kg

平口，直腹，圜底，立耳，柱足。礼器，祭祀器。

1965 年入藏。完整无损。

陕西医史博物馆藏

The tripod has a flat mouth, an erect belly, a round bottom, two prick ears, and three cylindrical legs. It used to be used as a sacrificial vessel. The tripod was collected in 1965 and is in good condition.

Preserved in Shaanxi Museum of Medical History

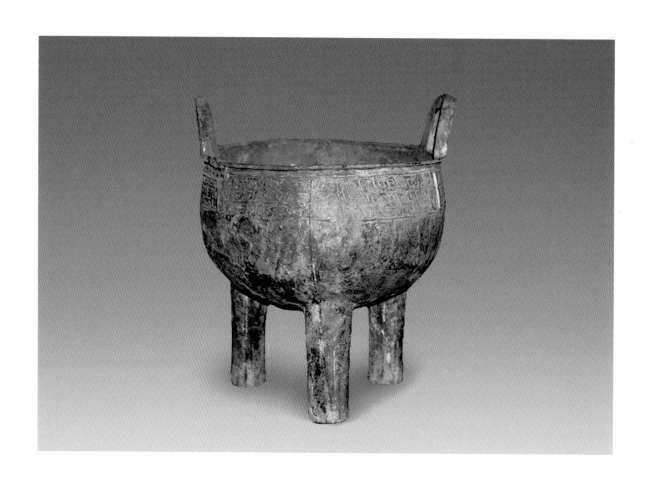

铜鼎

西周

青铜质

口径 20.5 厘米，通高 25 厘米，足高 10 厘米，重 2.9 千克

Bronze Tripod

Western Zhou Dynasty

Bronze

Mouth Diameter 20.5 cm/ Height 25 cm/ Height of the Leg 10 cm/ Weight 2.9 kg

平口沿，立耳，深腹，柱足。腹上夔纹。礼器。

陕西省咸阳市乾县征集。有残。

陕西医史博物馆藏

The tripod has a flat edge, prick ears, a deep belly and cylindrical legs. There is Kui dragon pattern on the belly. It used to be used as a sacrificial vessel. The tripod was collected from Qianxian County, Xianyang, Shaanxi Province. Part of it is damaged.

Preserved in Shaanxi Museum of Medical History

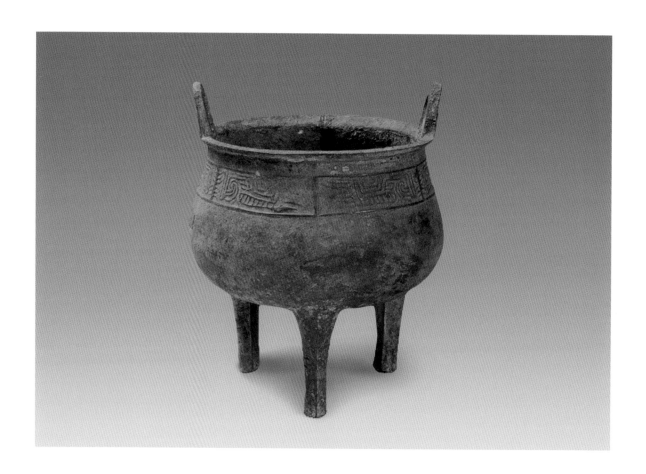

青铜变形饕餮纹鼎

西周

青铜质

通高 24.5 厘米

Bronze Tripod with Transformed Tao Tie Pattern

Western Zhou Dynasty

Bronze

Height 24.5 cm

立耳，垂腹，柱足。腹上部饰一周纹带，形似简化变形的饕餮纹，为饕餮正面相，以额鼻中线为界，身躯向两侧呈几形展开，其尾、足等处简化为排列整齐的短线，不施地纹，是以平行线条勾勒而成，显得较为纤弱，全无狰狞恐怖之感。溧水乌山岗沿山出土。

镇江博物馆藏

The tripod has prick ears, a vertical belly, and cylindrical legs. A circle of ribbon-like pattern is decorated on the upper belly. The pattern is similar in form of the front view of the simplified and transformed Tao Tie (a mythical ferocious animal) pattern, setting the forehead and nose as the center line, with its body spreading out to both sides like the shape of "几". The tail and feet, which are sketched with parallel lines, are simplified to neatly arranged short lines without setoff pattern. This design expresses the feeling of delicacy rather than ferociousness and horror. The tripod was unearthed Gangyan Mountain, Wushan Town, Lishui District.

Preserved in Zhenjiang Museum

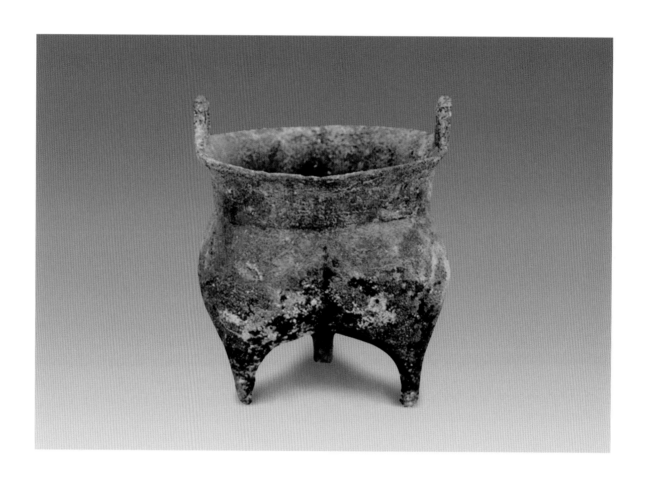

分裆鬲鼎

西周

青铜质

口径 14 厘米，通高 16.3 厘米

Li Tripod with Separated Crotch

Western Zhou Dynasty

Bronze

Mouth Diameter 14 cm/ Height 16.3 cm

立耳，侈口，束颈，分裆，鬲腹，大袋足。

颈饰一周雷纹带。1973 年山西省平陆县盘南

村出土。

山西博物院藏

The tripod has prick ears, a flare mouth, a narrowed neck, separated crotch and bellies, and bag-like legs. There is a circle of thunder pattern decorating the neck. The tripod was unearthed in Pannan Village, Pinglu County, Shanxi Province, in 1973.

Preserved in Shanxi Museum

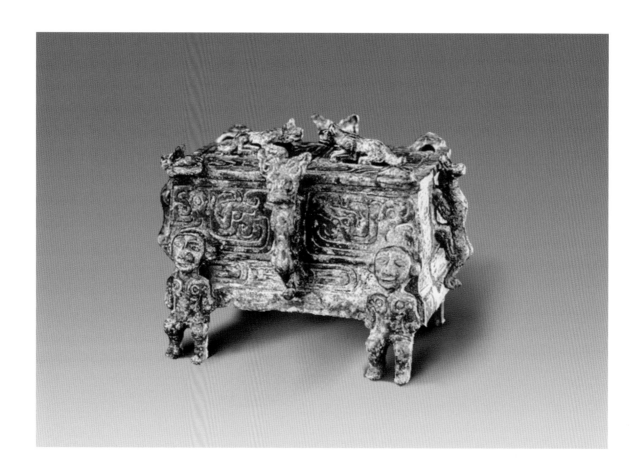

夔纹方鼎

西周

青铜质

长 9 厘米，宽 5.3 厘米，通高 8 厘米

Square Quadripod Ding with Kui Dragon Pattern

Western Zhou Dynasty

Bronze

Length 9 cm/ Width 5.3 cm/ Height 8 cm

器呈长方箱式，顶面双盖可启合，双盖上各
浮雕一伏虎，昂首竖耳，相互凝视，腹外四
壁中央竖雕龙、虎形，器下有四个奴隶人形
足，呈负器状。通体刻饰夔纹，制作精巧，
浮雕生动，是一个极有观赏价值的艺术珍品。
1974 年山西省闻喜县上郭村出土。

山西博物院藏

This is a rectangular box-like square quadripod.
The two covers of the quadripod can be opened
and closed, on which engraved are two prostrate
tigers looking at each other with their head
and ears up. Vertical dragons and tigers are
decorated in the center of the four outer walls
of the belly. Under the quadripod, there are four
slave-like feet carrying it. The whole quadripod
is engraved with exquisite Kui dragon pattern.
This quadripod is not only a lively design, but
also an art treasure of ornamental value. It was
unearthed in Shangguo Village, Wenxi County,
Shanxi Province, in 1974.

Preserved in Shanxi Museum

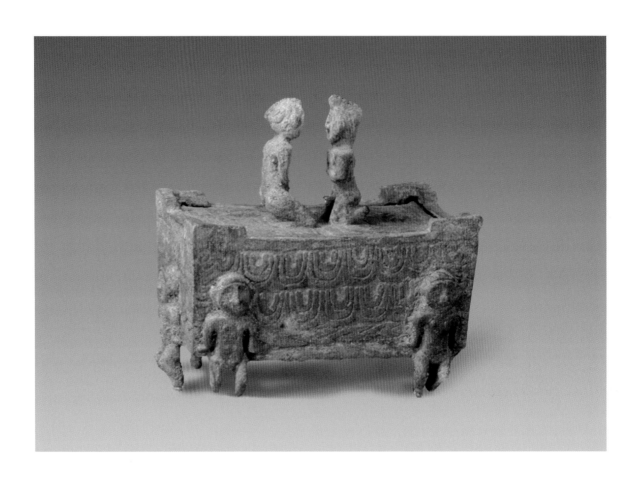

铜双人钮方鼎

西周

青铜质

长 11.2 厘米，宽 7.5 厘米，高 11.6 厘米

Square Quadripod with Two Man-like Figure Knobs

Western Zhou Dynasty

Bronze

Length 11.2 cm/ Width 7.5 cm/ Height 11.6 cm

长方形，有两盖，盖上有一对裸体相对跪坐
的男女形象，以六裸人为器足。

山东博物馆藏

There are two covers for this rectangular
cooking vessel, of which one has a naked man-
like design knob and the other has a woman-
like design kneeling face to face with each
other. Six naked man-like figures are designed
to serve as the feet of the vessel.
Preserved in Shandong Museum

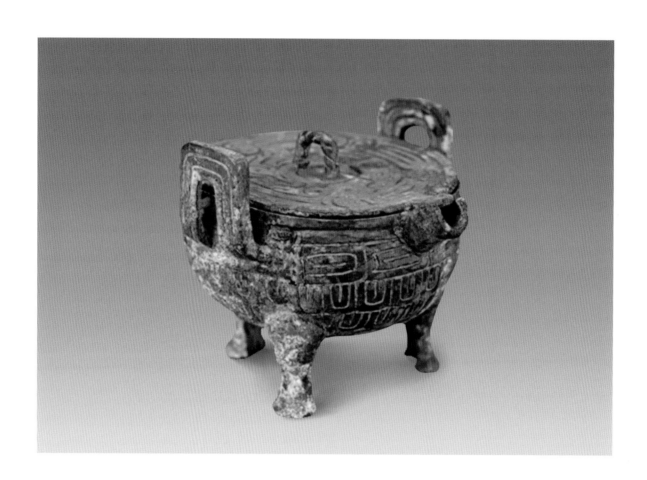

匜鼎

西周

青铜质

口径 8.8 厘米，通高 8 厘米

Tripod with a Ramp Spout

Western Zhou Dynasty

Bronze

Mouth Diameter 8.8 cm/ Height 8 cm

鼎口微敛，窄方唇，一侧呈匜形流。附耳，深腹，圆底，三蹄足。依口流形状设平盖，桥形方钮，饰扭索纹。盖面周边饰重环纹，内心饰窃曲纹，腹上部饰重环纹，下部饰垂鳞纹。

山西博物院藏

The tripod has a slightly small mouth, a narrow square lip, a ramp spout design on one side, two accessory ears, a deep belly, a round bottom, and three hoof-shaped feet. The flat cover of the tripod is designed according to the flow mouth, with a square bridge-like knob and guilloche decorated on it. Multiple layers of ring patterns are decorated not only around the surface of the cover but also on the upper belly, ragged curve is engraved in the center. The lower belly is decorated with hanging squama design.

Preserved in Shanxi Museum

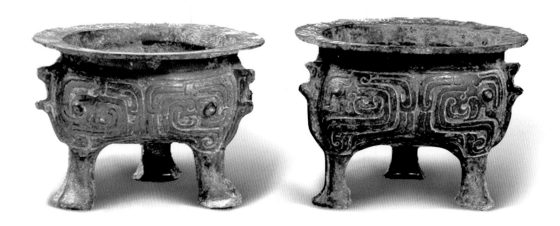

卫夫人鬲

西周

青铜质

口径 16 厘米，高 10.9 厘米

Li with Characters "Wei Fu Ren"

Western Zhou Dynasty

Bronze

Mouth Diameter 16 cm/ Height 10.9 cm

一对。宽平缘外折，束颈，圆肩，平裆，蹄足。腹饰扉棱，并有对称的卷体变形龙纹。两件鬲的口沿上均铸有铭文，共 28 字。

南京博物院藏

The two vessels have a big mouth, a wide flat rim that extends outward, a short neck, a round shoulder, a flat crotch, and hoof-like legs. On the belly, there are decorations of ridges, and coiling transformed dragon patterns in symmetry. The rim of the mouth of both vessels is cast with an inscription of 28 characters.

Preserved in Nanjing Museum

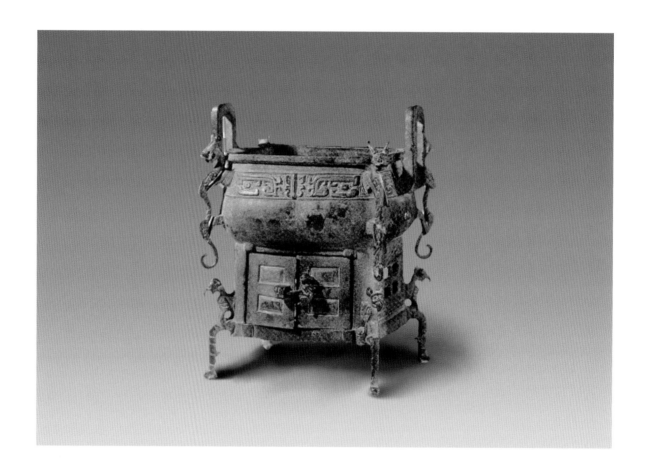

刖人守门方形青铜鬲

西周（前 1000—前 770)

青铜质

口径 11.9 厘米×9.2 厘米，通高 17.7 厘米

Square Bronze Li with a Yue Ren Guarding the Door

Western Zhou Dynasty (1000 B.C.–770 B.C.)

Bronze

Mouth Diameter 11.9 cm × 9.2 cm/ Height 17.7 cm

此件方形鬲口，鬲下四足间做成一封闭的房屋形，并铸出圆雕写实的人物形象，在已发现的商周青铜鬲中，这种造型与风格仅此一件。功能设计匠心独运，实用性与装饰性可谓完美结合。陕西省扶风县庄白窖藏出土。

陕西历史博物馆藏

This vessel has a square mouth. The lower part of the vessel over the four feet is made into a closed house in shape and cast with realistic figures in full relief. A Yue Ren is cast to guard the door. (Yue Ren refers to a man who was punished by cutting a foot or feet; cutting a man's foot or feet was a cruel punishment in the past in China). Among the bronze Li vessels of the Shang and Zhou Dynasties, this is the only unique one with such a modeling and style. The function and design of the vessel shows the designer's own ingenuity, which is a perfect combination of practical and decorative value. It was unearthed at Zhuangbai Village, Fufeng County, Shaanxi Province.

Preserved in Shaanxi History Museum

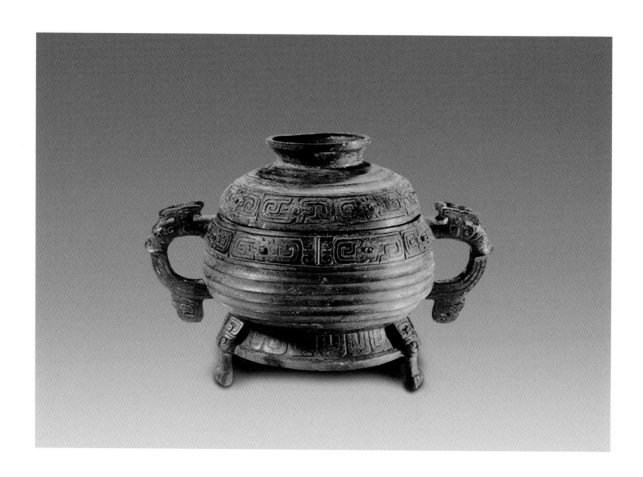

中再父簋

西周

青铜质

口径 21.5 厘米，通高 26.5 厘米

Gui with Characters "Zhong Chen Fu"

Western Zhou Dynasty

Bronze

Mouth Diameter 21.5 cm/ Height 26.5 cm

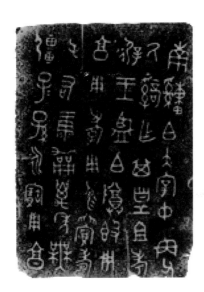

口微内敛，鼓腹。兽形双耳且带垂珥，微圜底，圈足外侈，下有三虎头矮足。上有盖，盖隆起，顶部有圆形捉手。通体用瓦纹、窃曲纹及垂鳞纹等装饰。器与盖对铭，铭文 44 字，系中国之相中再父为祭祀其祖、父两代人所作。食器。1981 年河南省南阳郊区砖瓦场出土。

河南博物院藏

The vessel has a swelling belly and a pair of handles in the shape of a beast with dropping decoration. The bottom of the vessel is slightly round in shape and the ring foot extends outward with three tiger-head shaped short feet under it. This vessel has a raised cover with a round knob handle on its top. The mouth of the vessel is slightly inwardly convergent. The whole body is decorated with the tile pattern, ragged curve and vertical scale pattern. The inscription of the cover corresponds with that of the body of the vessel, an inscription of 44 characters that say that this vessel was made by one of China's prime ministers as a sacrifice for his father and grandfather. This food container was unearthed from a tile field in the suburbs of Nanyang City of Henan Province.

Preserved in Henan Museum

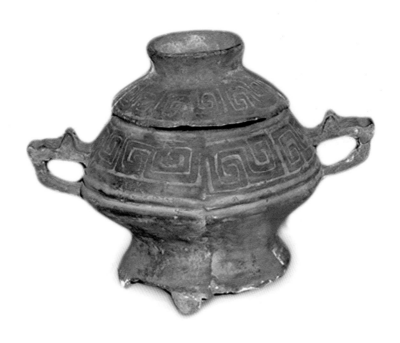

铜簋

西周

铜质

口径 9.3 厘米，底径 10.2 厘米，通高 13.5 厘米，重 1.15 千克

Copper Gui

Western Zhou Dynasty

Copper

Mouth Diameter 9.3 cm/ Bottom Diameter 10.2 cm/ Height 13.5 cm/ Weight 1.15 kg

束口，折腹。龙头双耳。饰有云雷纹，五足
残三。礼器，食器。三级文物。足有修补。
陕西省西安市鄠邑征集，20 世纪 70 年代入藏。

陕西医史博物馆藏

This food container has a convergent mouth,
a folded belly, and two dragon-head handles.
The vessel is decorated with cloud-thunder
pattern. There used to be five feet, but three
are damaged. This bronze Gui food container as
a grade Ⅲ cultural relic, and used as a sacrificial
and cooking vessel had its foot repaired. It was
collected from Huyi District, Xi'an City, Shaanxi
Province, and was collected in the museum in the
1970s.

Preserved in Shaanxi Museum of Medical History

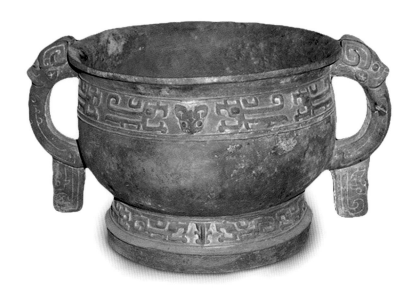

铜簋

西周

铜质

口径 22.1 厘米，底径 17.2 厘米，通高 16.2 厘米，重 3.1 千克

Copper Gui

Western Zhou Dynasty

Copper

Mouth Diameter 22.1 cm/ Bottom Diameter 17.2 cm/ Height 16.2 cm/ Weight 3.1 kg

鼓腹，圈足，双兽耳。上腹饰饕餮纹，底座
饰夔纹。礼器，盛贮器，二级文物。陕西省
咸阳市乾县征集。完整无损。

陕西医史博物馆藏

This vessel has a swelling belly, a ring foot and
two beast ears. Tao Tie pattern is engraved on
the upper belly, while Kui dragon pattern is
decorated on the pedestal. This food container,
which is in good condition, is a Grade II cultural
relic used as a sacrificial and food containing
vessel. It was collected from Qianxian County,
Xianyang City, Shaanxi Province.

Preserved in Shaanxi Museum of Medical History

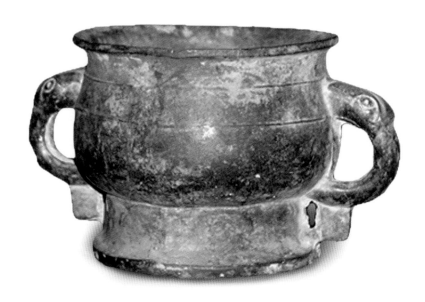

铜簋

西周（战国）

铜质

口径 15.6 厘米，底径 13.8 厘米，通高 12.7 厘米，重 2.1 千克

Copper Gui

Western Zhou Dynasty (the Warring States Period)

Copper

Mouth Diameter 15.6 cm/ Bottom Diameter 13.8 cm/ Height 12.7 cm/ Weight 2.1 kg

鼓腹，圈足，象鼻双耳。上腹有二道纹。礼器，生活用器，三级文物。底部有修补。陕西省兴平市征集。

陕西医史博物馆藏

This vessel has a swelling belly, a ring foot, and two ears in the shape of elephant nose. There are two streaks of pattern on the upper belly. This vessel had once its bottom repaired, and used to be used as a sacrificial vessel. It is a grade Ⅲ cultural relic. It was collected from Xingping City, Shaanxi Province.

Preserved in Shaanxi Museum of Medical History

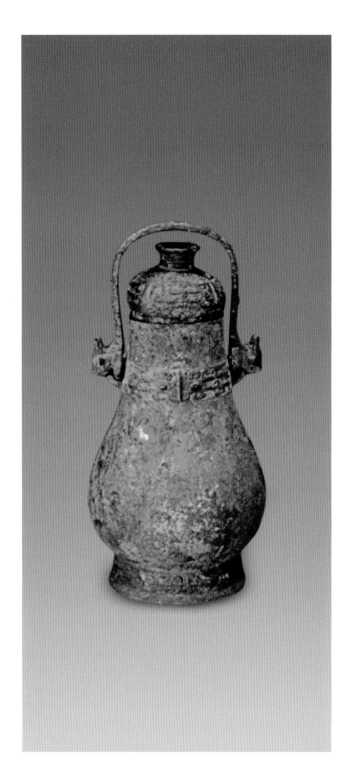

蠤父己卣

西周

青铜质

口径 9 厘米，底径 14.5 厘米，通高 37 厘米

You with Characters Including "蠤"

Western Zhou Dynasty

Bronze

Mouth Diameter 9 cm/ Bottom Diameter 14.5 cm/

Height 37 cm

器型细高，带状提梁，两端呈兽首状，盖呈
覆钵形，顶端有圈状捉手，直子口，鼓腹下垂，
高圈足。盖、足各饰雷纹地夔纹一周。盛酒器。

山西博物院藏

This vessel is slim and tall with a ribbon-
like hoop handle, both ends of which are cast
into the shape of an animal head. The cover is
shaped like an inverted alms bowl and on the
top of it is a ring knob. The ring convex of the
cover is straight and smaller than the mouth of
the vessel. The vessel has a drooping swelling
belly, and a high ring foot. The cover and the foot
are decorated with a band of whorled (thunder)
pattern and a band of Kui dragon pattern. This
vessel used to serve as a wine vessel.

Preserved in Shanxi Museum

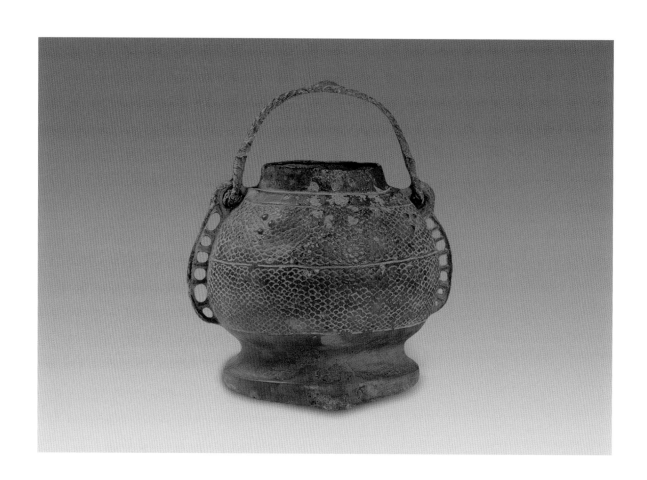

球腹鳞纹青铜卣

西周

青铜质

口径 15 厘米，腹径 27.6 厘米，通高 35 厘米

Bronze You with a Round Belly with Scale Patterns

Western Zhou Dynasty

Bronze

Mouth Diameter 15 cm/ Belly Diameter 27.6 cm/ Height 35 cm

直口，圆球形腹，圈足，腹两侧至肩部有扉
棱装饰，上接圆环耳。与两耳边接的提梁，
铸成弧形，两端套环连耳。腹部满饰细鳞纹，
肩的下部有两组左右对称的三颗乳钉，器体
比较厚重。南京市高淳区（原高淳县）漆桥
土墩墓出土。

高淳区文物管理委员会

This vessel has a straight mouth, a round belly,
and a ring foot. There are decorations of flanges
from the flanks of the belly to the shoulder
area and the flanges are connected with ring
ears linked with the arc-shaped hoop handle by
lantern rings. The belly is all decorated with fine
scale patterns. Under the shoulder there are two
symmetrical groups of three papilla designs.
The body is massive. It was excavated from the
Qiqiao Mound Tomb of Gaochun County.
Preserved in Gaochun Administration Committee
of Cultural Relics

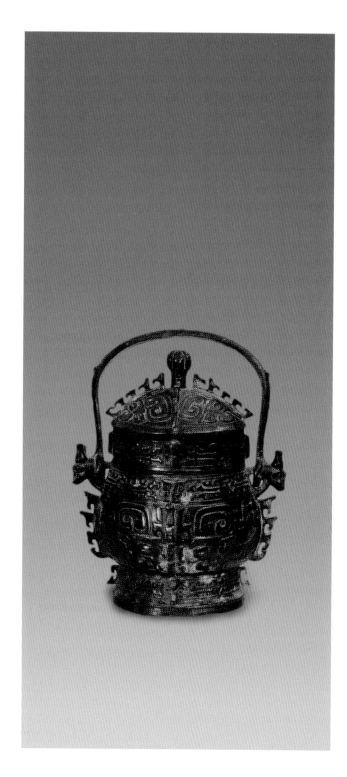

商卣

西周

青铜质

口径16.7厘米，腹深26.6厘米，高38.6厘米，

重 16.4 千克

You with Character "Shang"

Western Zhou Dynasty

Bronze

Mouth Diameter 16.7 cm/ Depth 26.6 cm/

Height 38.6 cm/ Weight 16.4 kg

四面扉棱，腹、盖饰饕餮纹，提梁两端有
兽头。容酒器。1976 年陕西扶风庄白一号
窖藏出土。

宝鸡市周原博物馆藏

There are flanges on the four sides of the
vessel with Tao Tie patterns on the belly
and the cover. There are designs of animal
heads on both ends of the hoop handle. This
vessel used to serve as a wine vessel and was
excavated from No.1 Zhuangbai Cellar of
Fufeng County, Shaanxi Province, in 1976.
Preserved in Zhouyuan Museum, Baoji City

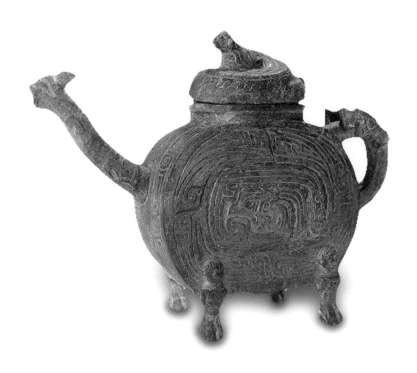

人形足兽首流盉

西周

青铜质

通长 30.3 厘米，高 22 厘米

He with Human-shaped Legs and Animal Head Shaped Spout

Wester Zhou Dynasty

Bronze

Width 30.3 cm/ Height 22 cm

扁圆腹，腹部外侧饰云纹，中心饰曲卷的龙纹。
直领小口上附盖，盖顶饰一曲躯的卧兽。细长
流，流口部为一张口的兽头。环形鋬上也有一
兽头装饰。腹下四足为裸体跪姿人形。1990 年
河南省三门峡虢国墓地 2001 号墓出土。

河南博物院藏

The belly of the vessel is flattened and circular in
shape decorated with cloud-like pattern outward and
curly dragon design in the center. There is a cover
on the small mouth, decorated with a beast curling up
on it. There is a narrow and long spout in the shape
of an open-mouth beast head design. There is
a beast-head design on the ring handle. The four
legs below the belly are in the shape of a naked
human kneeling down. In 1990, it was unearthed
in No. 2001 Guo Cemetery in Sanmenxia City,
Henan Province.

Preserved in Henan Museum

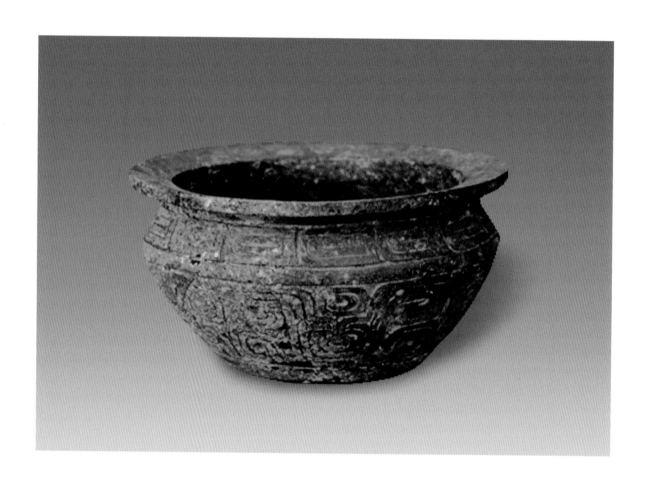

窃曲纹盂

西周

口径 19 厘米，通高 9.7 厘米

Yu with Qie Qu Pattern

Western Zhou Dynasty

Bronze

Mouth Diameter 19 cm/ Height 9.7 cm

敛口，宽斜折沿，圆折丰肩，斜壁，平底。
颈饰重环纹，腹饰窃曲纹，内填斜方格纹。

山西博物院藏

This ware has a convergent mouth, the edge of which is wide and oblique, and folded. The shoulder is big and round with a fold on it. The walls are titled and the bottom is flat. The neck is decorated with multiple rings pattern. The belly is decorated with Qie Qu pattern with oblique square pattern inside.

Preserved in Shanxi Museum

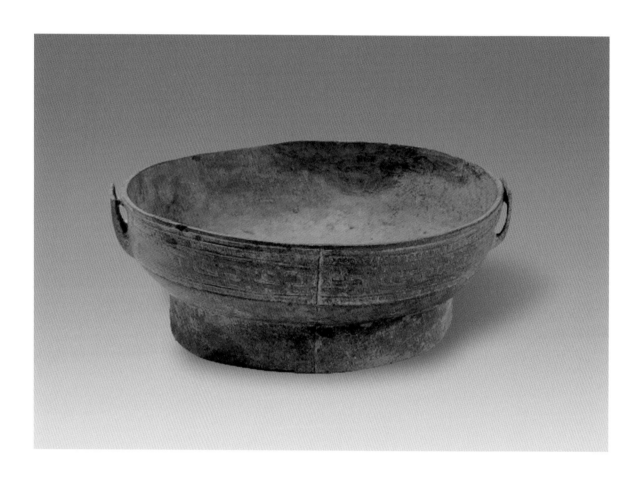

青铜夔纹盘

西周

青铜质

口径 30.3 厘米，底径 23.3 厘米，高 10.8 厘米

Bronze Plate with Kui Dragon Pattern

Western Zhou Dynasty

Bronze

Calibre 30.3 cm/ Bottom Diameter 23.3 cm/ Height 10.8 cm

直口，浅腹，圈足，双紧附耳与口沿平齐。盘腹饰夔纹，上下以圈点纹为边饰，圈足光素。此盘双耳作附耳，耳与器腹间仅容一指，已失去附耳功能，应是一种蜕化。这种现象在宁镇地区青铜盘类器上较多见，当属吴地青铜器的一种地方特色。溧水乌山岗沿山出土。

镇江博物馆藏

This plate has a straight mouth, a shallow belly, a ring foot and a pair of looped ears that are on the same level of the mouth. The belly is decorated with Kui dragon design, with punctuation pattern alongside the design. There is no pattern on the ring foot. The two ears on the belly are designed one-finger close to the wall, the function of which degenerated to decoration. Such a design approach is more commonly seen on the bronze plates produced in regions around Ningzhen Prefecture, and it represents the local characteristics of the bronze produced in Wu area. This plate was unearthed in Gangyan Hill of Mountain Wu in Lishui District.

Preserved in Zhenjiang Museum

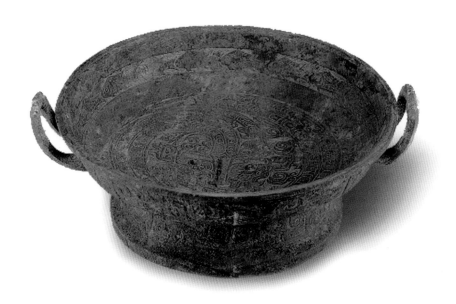

鱼龙纹铜盘

西周

青铜质

高 13 厘米

Bronze Plate with Stylized Dragon Design

Western Zhou Dynasty

Bronze

Height 13 cm

敞口外折，浅腹，平底，圈足外侈，两附耳
高出器口。口沿饰有弦纹和联珠纹，腹的外
壁与圈足部均饰夔纹一周，腹内壁有顺向鱼
纹一周。盘内底在鱼鳞纹地上饰有蟠龙纹。

河北博物院藏

There is an open mouth with edge folded
outward, a flat bottom, a ring foot folded
outward, and two ears protruding out of the
mouth. The edge of the mouth is decorated
with bowstring pattern and pattern of a string
of beads. Both the outer wall of the belly and
the ring foot are decorated with a circle of Kui
dragon pattern. The inner wall is decorated
clockwise with a circle of the pattern of fish.
The inner bottom is decorated with the pattern
of fish scale pattern, with curly dragon pattern
on the bottom layer.

Preserved in Hebei Museum

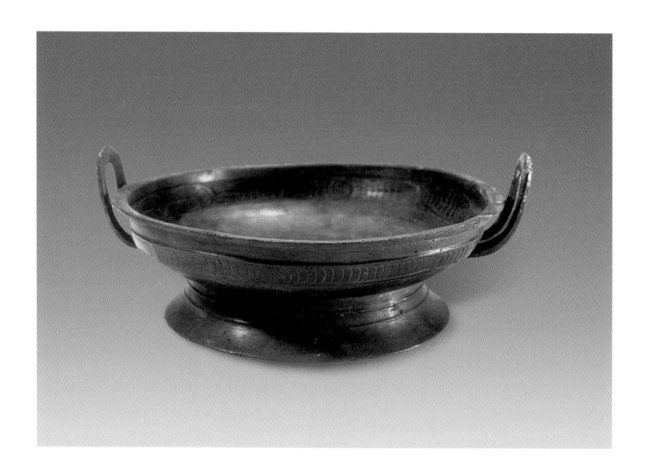

鱼龙纹盘

西周

青铜质

口径 27.5 厘米，通高 11.5 厘米

Plate with Stylized Dragon Design

Western Zhou Dynasty

Bronze

Calibre 27.5 cm/ Height 11.5 cm

敞口，平沿外折，浅腹，附耳，微圜底，圈
足外侈。盘外壁饰蛇纹、凸弦纹，内壁有鱼
纹一周，底部铸蟠龙纹。1981 年河南省南阳
郊区砖瓦厂出土。

河南博物院藏

There is an open mouth, a flat edge folded
outward, a shallow belly, two ears, a round
bottom, and a ring foot with edge folded
outward. The outer wall is decorated with snake
pattern and convex string pattern. The inner
wall is decorated with a circle of the pattern of
fish, with curly dragon pattern on the bottom.
In 1981, it was unearthed in a brick plant in the
suburbs of Nanyang City, Henan Province.
Preserved in Henan Museum

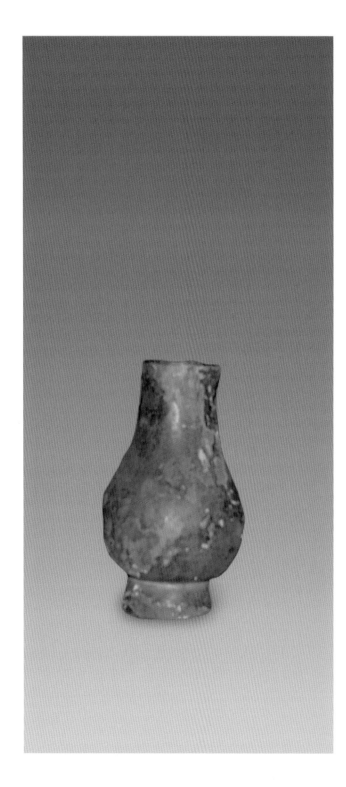

铜觯

西周

铜质

口径 4.5 厘米，底径 5.5 厘米，通高 13.4 厘米，
重 0.35 千克

Copper Zhi

Western Zhou Dynasty

Copper

Mouth Diameter 4.5 cm/ Bottom Diameter 5.5 cm/

Height 13.4 cm/ Weight 0.35 kg

直口，直颈，圆腹，倒喇叭形底座。酒器。

底残损。陕西省咸阳市废品站征集。

陕西医史博物馆藏

The vessel has a straight mouth, a straight
neck, a round belly, and an inverted trumpet-
like pedestal. It was used as a drinking vessel.
The pedestal is incomplete. It was collected
in a salvage point in Xianyang City, Shaanxi
Province.

Preserved in Shaanxi Museum of Medical History

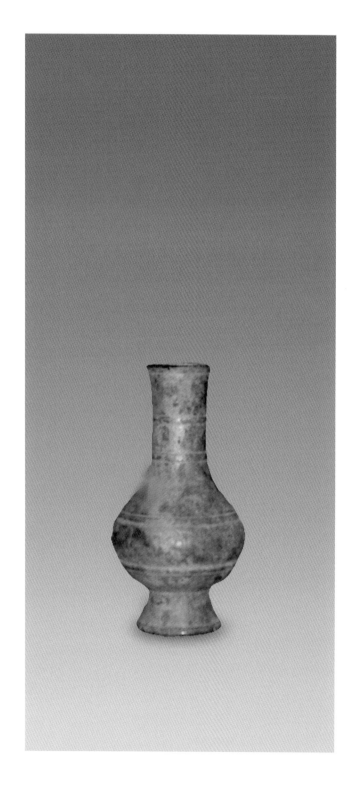

铜觯

西周

铜质

口径4.4厘米，底径5.8厘米，通高17.5厘米，
重 0.6 千克

Copper Zhi

Western Zhou Dynasty

Copper

Mouth Diameter 4.4cm/ Bottom Diameter 5.8cm/

Height 17.5cm/ Weight 0.6 kg

圆口，直颈，鼓腹，倒喇叭形底座。酒器。

三级文物。完整无损。陕西省咸阳市废品站

征集，20 世纪 70 年代入藏。

陕西医史博物馆藏

The vessel has a round mouth, a straight neck, a swelling belly, and an inverted trumpet-like pedestal. It was used as a drinking vessel. It is a grade Ⅲ cultural relic at the national level. The vessel is intact good condtion. It was collected in a salvage point in Xianyang City, Shaanxi Province. The vessel was collected in the 1970's. Preserved in Shaanxi Museum of Medicine History

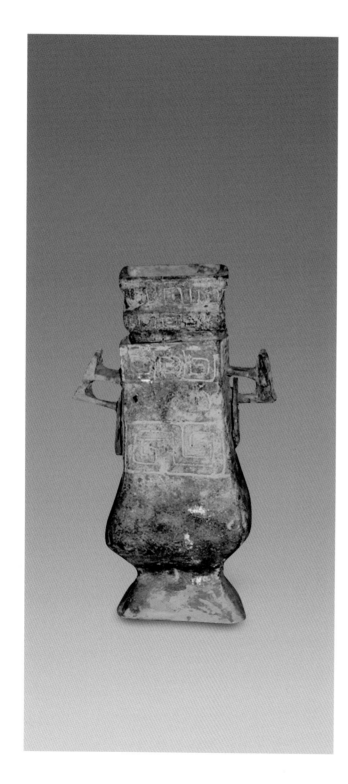

铜方壶

西周

铜质

口径 6.2 厘米，底径 8.5 厘米，通高 22 厘米，
重 1.4 千克

Square Copper Pot

Western Zhou Dynasty

Copper

Mouth Diameter 6.2 cm/ Bottom Diameter 8.5 cm/

Height 22 cm/ Weight 1.4 kg

子母口，方垂腹，双兽耳，耳上各套一环，
腹上饰雷纹，方形底座。酒器。完整无损。
陕西省西安市鄠邑区征集。

陕西医史博物馆藏

The pot has a snap-lid cover, a square and drooping belly, and two ears in the shape of a beast head with a hitched ring. The belly is decorated with thunder pattern. There is a square pedestal. The pot was used as a drinking vessel. The pot is intact in shape. The relic was collected in Huyi District, Xi'an City, Shaanxi Province.

Preserved in Shaanxi Museum of Medical History

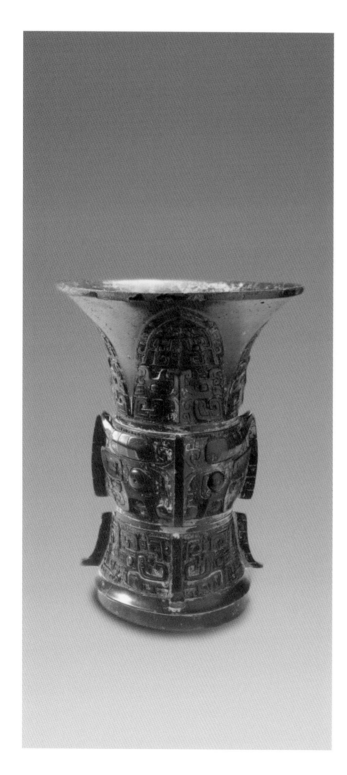

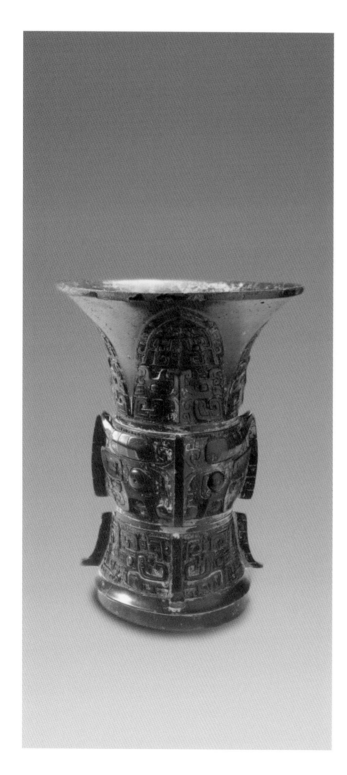（食）尊

西周

青铜质

口径 21.8 厘米，高 28.3 厘米

Zun with Character "" (Shi)

Western Zhou Dynasty

Bronze

Mouth Diameter 21.8 cm/ Height 28.3 cm

侈口，长颈，微鼓腹，圜底，高圈足略外侈。颈部以四组大蕉叶纹装饰；腹部与圈足有四条突起的扉棱，并饰有两组用雷纹为底的饕餮纹，且饕餮的眉、目浮起，突出外。圈足内铭一"𩜹"（食）字。1985 年河南省济源下冶乡（今下冶镇）出土。

河南博物院藏

The vessel has a flared mouth, a long neck, a relatively swelling belly, a round bottom, and a tall ring foot that slightly protrudes outward. The neck is decorated with four groups of plantain leaves patterns. There are four protuberant ridges on the belly and the ring foot which are decorated with Tao Tie pattern. Tao Tie has protruding eyes and eyebrows. The interior ring foot is inscribed with a character "𩜹" (Shi). The vessel was unearthed in Xiaye County (now Xiaye Town), Jiyuan City, Henan Province, in 1985.

Preserved in Henan Museum

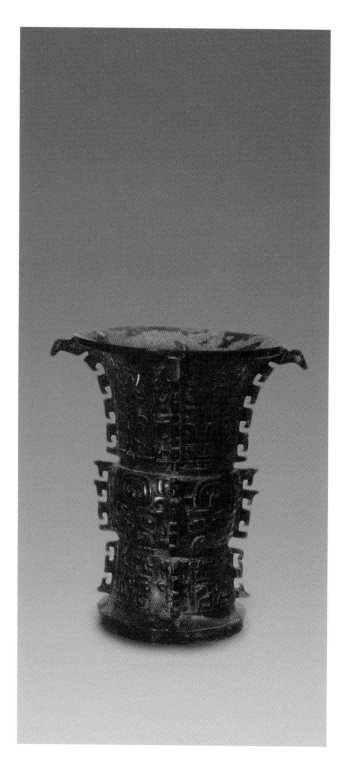

商尊

西周

青铜质

口径23.6厘米，腹深22.9厘米，通高30.4厘米，
重 11.7 千克

Zun with Character "Shang"

Western Zhou Dynasty

Bronze

Mouth Diameter 23.6 cm/ Depth 22.9 cm/

Height 30.4 cm/ Weight 11.7 kg

四周有扉棱，腹有饕餮纹，颈有龙纹。腹底有 3 行 30 字铭文。盛酒器。1976 年陕西扶风周原庄白一号窖藏出土。

宝鸡市周原博物馆藏

The vessel has ridges around its body, Tao Tie pattern on the belly and a dragon design on the neck. There is an inscription of 30 characters in 3 lines on the bottom of the belly. It served as a wine vessel. The vessel was unearthed in No. 1 cellar in Zhouyuan Village, Fufeng County, Shaanxi Province, in 1976.

Preserved in Zhouyuan Museum, Baoji City

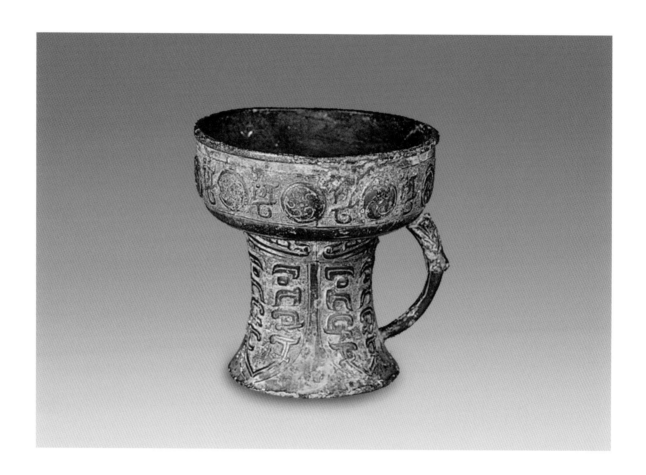

康生豆

西周

青铜质

口径 15 厘米，通高 14.5 厘米

Dou with Characters "Kang Sheng"

Western Zhou Dynasty

Bronze

Mouth Diameter 15 cm/ Height 14.5 cm

盘呈深腹平底，口微敛，唇边凸起，下承喇
叭形高圈足，腹足间一侧置兽首形曲柄。通
体以雷纹衬地，盘腹饰一周圆涡纹，间饰回
首夔纹；足上部饰一周夔纹，下垂四组蕉叶
纹，间饰兽面纹。

山西博物院藏

The container has a deep belly and a flat
bottom. The mouth is convergent, and the
edge of lip is bulged. There is a long trumpet-
shaped ring foot, and an animal head-shaped
crank between the belly and the foot. The whole
body is decorated with thunder patterns as the
ground-tint. Then, there is a circle of round
vortex pattern on the belly, within the pattern,
there is a Kui dragon pattern turning back its
head. There is a circle of Kui dragon pattern on
the upper foot, and four-group of plantain leaf-
like patterns drooping down, within it there is
beast face pattern inside it.

Preserved in Shanxi Museum

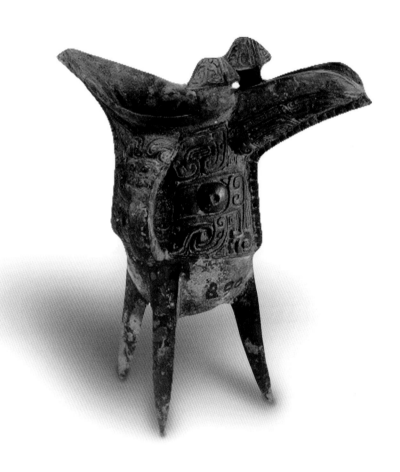

亚又口爵

西周

青铜质

口宽 8 厘米，高 20.7 厘米

Jue with Characters "Ya You Kou"

West Zhou Dynasty

Bronze

Mouth Width 8cm/ Height 20.7cm

爵形，三足，两柱。两柱顶为四阿房形，腹高浮雕饕餮纹，内有"亚又口"三字。温饮酒器。陕西淳化黑豆嘴出土。

淳化县文博馆藏

This is a three-footed vessel with two columns and the upper part of the bady is decorated with ogre mask motif in relief. There is an inscription of "Ya You Kou" inside. This is a vessel for keeping wine warm. It was unearthed in Heidouzui of Chunhua County, Shaanxi Province.

Preserved in Chunhua County Museum

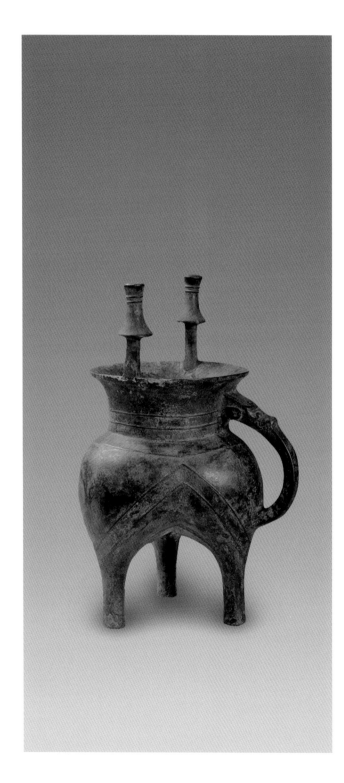

铜斝

西周

青铜质

口径 15.6 厘米，通高 31.5 厘米

Bronze Jia

West Zhou Dynasty

Bronze

Diameter 15.6 cm/ Height 31.5 cm

侈口，沿上有伞形双柱，把上饰兽面纹。腹
呈袋形，分裆，下有三长柱形足。颈部饰两
周弦纹，腹部饰弦纹及双线人字纹。把内的
腹上铸有铭文。

南京市博物馆藏

This vessel has a flared mouth, with two columns
in the shape of an umbrella on its edge. The
handle is decorated with animal mask pattern,
and the belly is shaped like a bag. The body of the
vessel is supported by long cylindrical tripodal
legs. The neck is decorated with two circles of
bowstring patterns while the belly is decorated
with bowstring patterns and double-line zigzag
patterns. The inscription is on the inner side of
the handle.

Preserved in Nanjing Municipal Museum

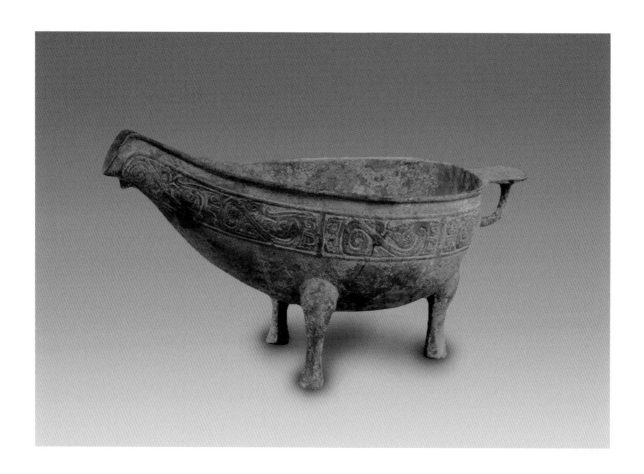

铜匜

西周

铜质

长 39.2 厘米，通高 21.2 厘米

Copper Yi

Western Zhou Dynasty

Copper

Length 39.2 cm/ Height 21.2 cm

器形如瓢，无盖，折沿，腹身较扁长，圜底，
下具三蹄足。流部下方有一小支钉，呈凤尾
状。两侧腹部饰同向的回顾龙纹，尾錾饰弧
曲雷纹与卷云状的羽纹。

南京市博物馆藏

The bronze artifact is in the shape of ladle
without a cover and with folded edges. It has a
long flattened belly and a round bottom which is
supported by tripodal legs in hoof-shape. Under
the spout, there is a small support pin, shaped
like the tail of a phoenix. The two sides of the
belly are decorated with patterns of dragons,
both looking back in the same direction. The
handle is decorated with the bent string thunder
patterns and feather patterns in cirrus clouds.
Preserved in Nanjing Municipal Museum

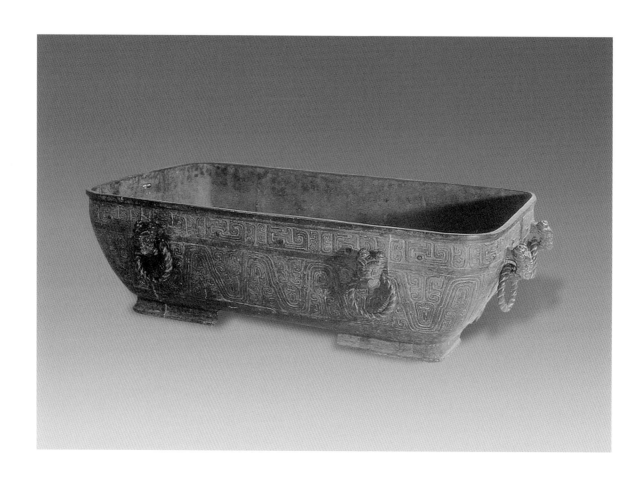

虢季子白盘

西周

青铜质

长 130.2 厘米，宽 82.7 厘米，高 41.3 厘米

Plate with Characters "Guo Ji Zi Bai"

Western Zhou Dynasty

Bronze

Length 130.2 cm/ Width 82.7 cm/ Height 41.3 cm

长方形，有铭文 111 字。为传世最大的西周
时代青铜器。可用于洗浴。清道光年间于陕
西宝鸡虢川司出土。

中国国家博物馆藏

The plate is rectangular with an inscription of 111
characters. It is the biggest bronze ware in Western
Zhou Dynasty that has ever been discovered at
present. It could be used for bathing. It was
excavated in Guochuansi of Baoji City, Shaanxi
Province, in the reign of Emperor Daoguang of
the Qing Dynasty.

Preserved in National Museum of China

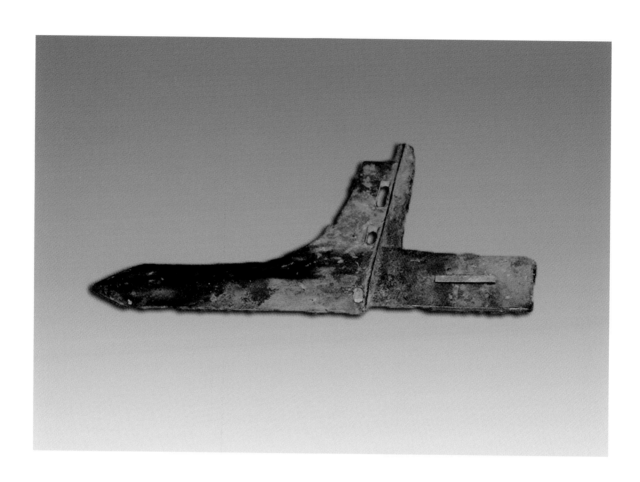

铜戈

西周

铜质

长 18 厘米，宽 11 厘米，底径 3 厘米，重 250 克

Copper Dagger-axe

Western Zhou Dynasty

Copper

Length 18 cm/ Width 11 cm/ Bottom Diameter 3 cm/ Weight 250 g

兵器。柄前端呈匕首状，中间有一棱，柄端
有三个长方形孔，柄为长方形，柄中间镂空。
完整无损。

陕西医史博物馆藏

The dagger-axe was a weapon. The front end
of the hilt is in the shape of a dagger with a ridge
in the middle. The rear end of the hilt is in the
shape of a hollow rectangle with three rectangular
apertures. It is intact and undamaged.

Preserved in Shaanxi Museum of Medical History

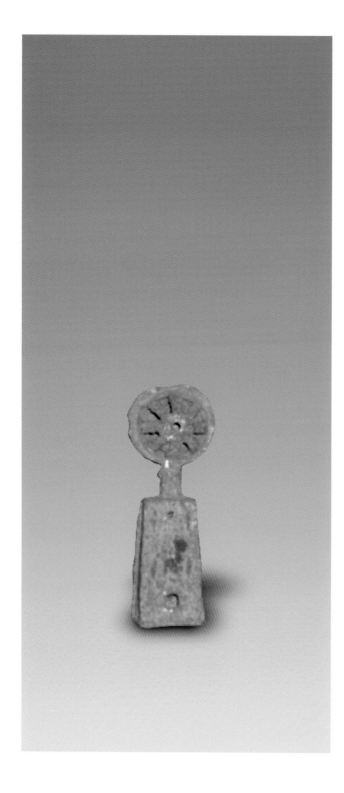

铜铃

西周

铜质

口径 5.5 厘米，通高 13.5 厘米，底径 3.5 厘米，
重 750 克

Copper Bell

West Zhou dynasty

Copper

Diameter 5.5 cm/ Height 13.5 cm/ Bottom
Diameter 3.5 cm/ Weight 750 g

上为一风扇形铃，下为长方形座，下腹四侧
各有一孔。车饰。完整无损。陕西省咸阳市
废品站征集。

陕西医史博物馆藏

This bell, intact and undamaged, is a decorative
part for carriage. There is a fan-shaped bell
at the upper part and a rectangle base at the
bottom with a hole in four sides respectively. It
was collected from a junk station in Xianyang
City, Shaanxi Province.

Preserved in Shaanxi Museum of Medical History

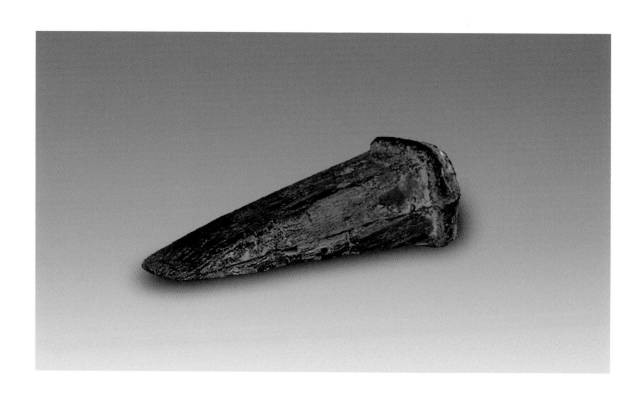

铜斧

西周

铜质

长 12 厘米，宽 3.5 厘米，底径 4 厘米，重 400 克

斧状，底有一方孔。生产工具。完整无损。

陕西医史博物馆藏

Copper Axe

Western Zhou dynasty

Copper

Length 12 cm/ Width 3.5 cm/ Bottom Diameter 4 cm/
Weight 400 g

The bronze relic is hatchet-shaped with a square hole at the bottom. It has been used as a labor too. It is still in good condition.

Preserved in Shaanxi Museum of Medical History

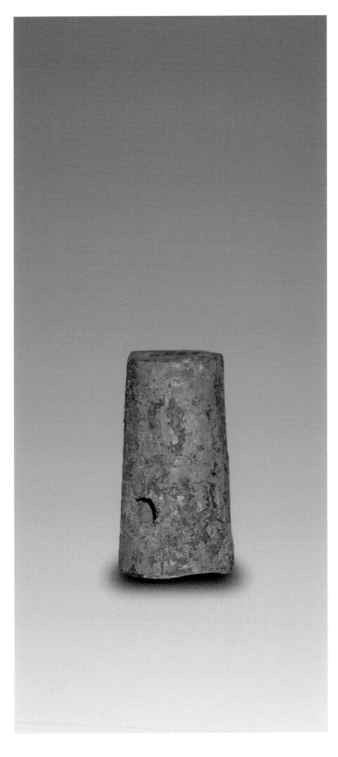

铜车饰

周

铜质

口径 3.7 米，通高 8 厘米，底径 4.3 厘米，
重 150 克

直筒状，周身夔纹，下腹有对称两小孔。车饰。
完整无损。

陕西医史博物馆藏

Copper Carriage Decoration

Zhou dynasty

Copper

Diameter 3.7 m/ Height 8 cm/ Bottom Diameter
4.3 cm/ Weight 150 g

This collection is a decorative component for
carriage. It is in the shape of a straight tube with
a hole symmetrically at the bottom bell part and
covered with Kui dragon pattern, a unique animal
motif pattern in ancient China. It is undamaged.

Preserved in Shaanxi Museum of Medical History

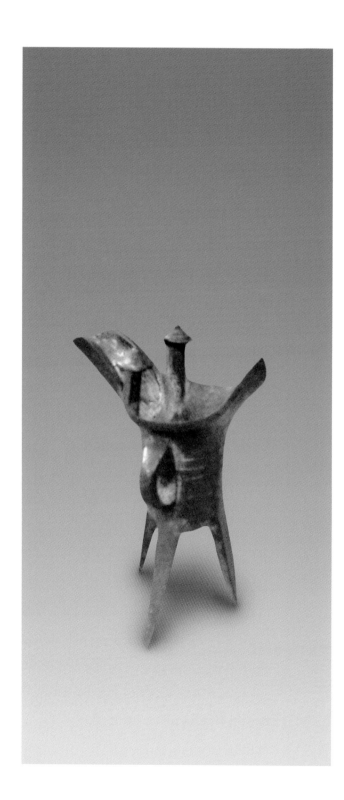

铜爵

周

铜

口径 12.2 厘米，通高 17.6 厘米

Copper Jue

Zhou Dynasty

Copper

Mouth Diameter 12.2 cm/ Height 17.6 cm

爵形，三足，两柱，带流，桥形耳。爵身有
三弦纹。造型美观，表面粗糙，为复制品。
饮酒器。保存基本完好。1960 年入藏。

中华医学会 / 上海中医药大学医史博物馆藏

The vessel has tripodal feet, two columns, a
spout and a bridge-like handle. The body of the
vessel has three belts of string pattern, The vessel
has an attractive design though the appearance is
rough. It was a replica of the original, and served as a
vessel for drinking wine. It was collected in 1960 and
is still in good condition.

Preserved in Chinese Medical Association/ Museum
of Chinese Medicine, Shanghai University of
Traditional Chinese Medicine

索 引

（馆藏地按拼音字母排序）

Index

参考文献

[1] 李经纬. 中国古代医史图录 [M]. 北京：人民卫生出版社，1992.

[2] 傅维康，李经纬，林昭庚. 中国医学通史：文物图谱卷 [M]. 北京：人民卫生出版社，2000.

[3] 和中浚，吴鸿洲. 中华医学文物图集 [M]. 成都：四川人民出版社，2001.

[4] 上海中医药博物馆. 上海中医药博物馆馆藏珍品 [M]. 上海：上海科学技术出版社，2013.

[5] 西藏自治区博物馆. 西藏博物馆 [M]. 北京：五洲传播出版社，2005.

[6] 崔乐泉. 中国古代体育文物图录：中英文本 [M]. 北京：中华书局，2000.

[7] 张金明，陆雪春. 中国古铜镜鉴赏图录 [M]. 北京：中国民族摄影艺术出版社，2002.

[8] 文物精华编辑委员会. 文物精华 [M]. 北京：文物出版社，1964.

[9] 谭维四. 湖北出土文物精华 [M]. 武汉：湖北教育出版社，2001.

[10] 常州市博物馆. 常州文物精华 [M]. 北京：文物出版社，1998.

[11] 镇江博物馆. 镇江文物精华 [M]. 合肥：黄山书社，1997.

[12] 贵州省文化厅，贵州省博物馆. 贵州文物精华 [M]. 贵阳：贵州人民出版社，2005.

[13] 徐良玉. 扬州馆藏文物精华 [M]. 南京：江苏古籍出版社，2001.

[14] 昭陵博物馆，陕西历史博物馆. 昭陵文物精华 [M]. 西安：陕西人民美术出版社，1991.

[15] 南通博物苑. 南通博物苑文物精华 [M]. 北京：文物出版社，2005.

[16] 邯郸市文物研究所. 邯郸文物精华 [M]. 北京：文物出版社，2005.

[17] 张秀生，刘友恒，聂连顺，等. 中国河北正定文物精华 [M]. 北京：文化艺术出版社，1998.

[18] 陕西省咸阳市文物局. 咸阳文物精华 [M]. 北京：文物出版社，2002.

[19] 安阳市文物管理局. 安阳文物精华 [M]. 北京：文物出版社，2004.

[20] 深圳市博物馆. 深圳市博物馆文物精华 [M]. 北京：文物出版社，1998.

[21]《中国文物精华》编辑委员会. 中国文物精华（1993）[M]. 北京：文物出版社，1993.

[22] 夏路，刘永生.山西省博物馆馆藏文物精华 [M].太原：山西人民出版社，1999.

[23] 文物精华编辑委员会.文物精华 [M].北京：文物出版社，1957.

[24] 山西博物院，湖北省博物馆.荆楚长歌：九连墩楚墓出土文物精华 [M].太原：山西人民出版社，2011.

[25] 刘广堂，石金鸣，宋建忠.晋国雄风：山西出土两周文物精华 [M].沈阳：万卷出版公司，2009.

[26] 沈君山，王国平，单迎红.滦平博物馆馆藏文物精华 [M].北京：中国文联出版社，2012.

[27] 张家口市博物馆.张家口市博物馆馆藏文物精华 [M].北京：科学出版社，2011.

[28] 浙江省文物考古研究所.浙江考古精华 [M].北京：文物出版社，1999.

[29] 故宫博物院.故宫雕刻珍萃 [M].北京：紫禁城出版社，2004.

[30] 故宫博物院紫禁城出版社.故宫博物院藏宝录 [M].上海：上海文艺出版社，1986.

[31] 首都博物馆.大元三都 [M].北京：科学出版社，2016.

[32] 新疆维吾尔自治区博物馆.新疆出土文物 [M].北京：文物出版社，1975.

[33] 王兴伊，段逸山.新疆出土涉医文书辑校 [M].上海：上海科学技术出版社，2016.

[34] 刘学春.刍议医药卫生文物的概念与分类标准 [J].中华中医药杂志，2016，31（11）:4406-4409.

[35] 上海古籍出版社.中国艺海 [M].上海：上海古籍出版社，1994.

[36] 紫都，岳鑫.一生必知的 200 件国宝 [M].呼和浩特：远方出版社，2005.

[37] 谭维四.湖北出土文物精华 [M].武汉：湖北教育出版社，2001.

[38] 张建青.青海彩陶收藏与鉴赏 [M].北京：中国文史出版社，2007.

[39] 银景琦.仡佬族文物 [M].南宁：广西人民出版社，2014.

[40] 廖果，梁峻，李经纬.东西方医学的反思与前瞻 [M].北京：中医古籍出版社，2002.

[41] 梁峻，张志斌，廖果，等.中华医药文明史集论 [M].北京：中医古籍出版社，2003.

[42] 郑蓉，庄乾竹，刘聪，等.中国医药文化遗产考论 [M].北京：中医古籍出版社，2005.